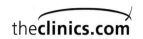

SURGICAL CLINICS
OF NORTH AMERICA

Surgery as an Industry: Evolution or Revolution?

GUEST EDITORS
Ronald F. Martin, MD
Vijay P. Khatri, MBChB, FACS

CONSULTING EDITOR
Ronald F. Martin, MD

August 2007 • Volume 87 • Number 4

SAUNDERS

An Imprint of Elsevier, Inc.
PHILADELPHIA   LONDON   TORONTO   MONTREAL   SYDNEY   TOKYO

W.B. SAUNDERS COMPANY
A Division of Elsevier Inc.

1600 John F. Kennedy Blvd., Suite 1800, Philadelphia, PA 19103-2899

http://www.theclinics.com

SURGICAL CLINICS OF NORTH AMERICA
August 2007
Editor: Catherine Bewick

Volume 87, Number 4
ISSN 0039–6109
ISBN-10: 1-4160-5125-2
ISBN-13: 978-1-4160-5125-1

The ideas and opinions expressed in *The Surgical Clinics of North America* do not necessarily reflect those of the Publisher. The Publisher does not assume any responsibility for any injury and/or damage to persons or property arising out of or related to any use of the material contained in this periodical. The reader is advised to check the appropriate medical literature and the product information currently provided by the manufacturer of each drug to be administered to verify the dosage, the method and duration of administration, or contraindications. It is the responsibility of the treating physician or other health care professional, relying on independent experience and knowledge of the patient, to determine drug dosages and the best treatment for the patient. Mention of any product in this issue should not be construed as endorsement by the contributors, editors, or the Publisher of the product or manufacturers' claims.

Surgical Clinics of North America (ISSN 0039–6109) is published bimonthly by Elsevier Inc., 360 Park Avenue South, New York, NY 10010-1710. Months of publication are February, April, June, August, October, and December. Business and Editorial Offices: 1600 John F. Kennedy Blvd., Suite 1800, Philadelphia, PA 19103-2899. Customer Service Office: 6277 Sea Harbor Drive, Orlando, FL 32887-4800. Periodicals postage paid at New York, NY and additional mailing offices. Subscription prices are $220.00 per year for US individuals, $347.00 per year for US institutions, $110.00 per year for US students and residents, $270.00 per year for Canadian individuals, $424.00 per year for Canadian institutions, $286.00 for international individuals, $424.00 per year for international institutions and $143.00 per year for Canadian and foreign students/residents. To receive student/resident rate, orders must be accompanied by name of affiliated institution, date of term, and the *signature* of program/residency coordinator on institution letterhead. Orders will be billed at individual rate until proof of status is received. Foreign air speed delivery is included in all *Clinics* subscription prices. All prices are subject to change without notice. POSTMASTER: Send address changes to *Surgical Clinics*, Elsevier Periodicals Customer Service, 6277 Sea Harbor Drive, Orlando, FL 32887-4800. **Customer Service: 1-800-654-2452 (US). From outside of the US, call 1-407-345-1000.**

The Surgical Clinics of North America is also published in Spanish by McGraw-Hill Interamericana Editores S.A., P.O. Box 5-237 06500 Mexico D.F. Mexico; and in Portuguese by Interlivros Edicoes Ltda., Rua Comandante Coelho 1085, CEP 21250, Rio de Janeiro, Brazil; and in Greek by Paschalidis Medical Publications, Athens Greece.

The Surgical Clinics of North America is covered in *Index Medicus, EMBASE/Excerpta Medica, Current Contents/Clinical Medicine, Current Contents/Life Sciences, Science Citation Index,* and *ISI/BIOMED.*

Printed in the United States of America.

CONSULTING EDITOR

RONALD F. MARTIN, MD, Staff Surgeon, Marshfield Clinic, Marshfield, Wisconsin; Lieutenant Colonel, Medical Corps, United States Army Reserve

GUEST EDITORS

RONALD F. MARTIN, MD, Staff Surgeon, Marshfield Clinic, Marshfield, Wisconsin; Lieutenant Colonel, Medical Corps, United States Army Reserve

VIJAY P. KHATRI, MBChB, FACS, Professor of Surgery, Division of Surgical Oncology, University of California, Davis Cancer Center, Sacramento, California

CONTRIBUTORS

MELISSA B. BANKER, BA, Education Project Coordinator, American Board of Surgery, Philadelphia, Pennsylvania

RICHARD H. BELL, JR, MD, Assistant Executive Director, American Board of Surgery, Philadelphia, Pennsylvania

THOMAS W. BIESTER, MS, Director of Psychometrics and Data Analysis, American Board of Surgery, Philadelphia, Pennsylvania

DARRELL C. CAMPBELL, JR, MD, Professor of Surgery, Chief of Clinical Affairs, The University of Michigan Hospitals and Health Centers, Ann Arbor, Michigan

KATHLEEN M. CASEY, MD, FACS, Director, Operation Giving Back, American College of Surgeons, Chicago, Illinois

ANDREW B. COOPER, MD, MHSc, The Interdisciplinary Division of Critical Care Medicine, University of Toronto, Toronto; Sunnybrook and Women's College Health Sciences Centre, Toronto, Ontario, Canada

SUZANNE DELBANCO, PhD, Chief Executive Officer, The Leapfrog Group, Washington, DC

AARON S. FINK, MD, Professor of Surgery, Emory University School of Medicine; Manager, Surgical and Perioperative Care, Veterans Administration Medical Center–Atlanta, Decatur, Georgia

KAMAL M. ITANI, MD, Professor of Surgery, Boston University School of Medicine; Associate Chief of Surgery for Veterans Affairs, Boston Medical Center and Brigham and Women's Hospitals; Chief, Surgical Service, Veterans Administration Boston Healthcare System, Boston, Mssachusetts

JAY A. JACOBSON, MD, FACP, Chief, Division of Medical Ethics and Humanities Member, Division of Infectious Diseases, Departments of Internal Medicine, LDS Hospital and the University of Utah School of Medicine, Salt Lake City, Utah

LAURANCE JERROLD, DDS, JD, ABO, Orthodontist; Attorney; Bioethicist; Dean and Program Director, School of Orthodontics, Jacksonville University, Jacksonville, Florida

JAMES W. JONES, MD, PhD, MHA, Montgomery, Texas

FRANK R. LEWIS, MD, Executive Director, American Board of Surgery, Philadelphia, Pennsylvania

MICHAEL H. McCAFFERTY, MD, Associate Professor, Department of Surgery, University of Louisville, Louisville, Kentucky

LAWRENCE B. McCULLOUGH, PhD, Center for Medical Ethics and Health Policy, Baylor College of Medicine, Houston, Texas

MARTIN McKNEALLY, MD, PhD, Joint Centre for Bioethics, University of Toronto, Toronto, Ontario, Canada

HIRAM C. POLK, JR, MD, Ben A. Reid, Senior Professor, Department of Surgery, University of Louisville, Louisville, Kentucky

SHARON REYNOLDS, RN, BA, BScN, MHSc, Joint Centre for Bioethics, University of Toronto, Toronto, Ontario; Medical-Surgical Intensive Care Unit, Toronto General Hospital, Toronto, Ontario, Canada

BRUCE W. RICHMAN, MA, Columbia, Missouri

ROBERT S. RHODES, MD, Adjunct Professor, Department of Surgery, University of Pennsylvania School of Medicine, Philadelphia; Associate Executive Director and Director of Evaluation, American Board of Surgery, Philadelphia, Pennsylvania

THOMAS R. RUSSELL, MD, FACS, Executive Director, American College of Surgeons, Chicago, Illinois

AJIT K. SACHDEVA, MD, FRCSC, FACS, Director, Division of Education, American College of Surgeons, Chicago, Illinois

CONTENTS

Foreword xi
Ronald F. Martin

Preface xv
Ronald F. Martin and Vijay P. Khatri

The Surgical Workforce: Averting a Patient Access Crisis 797
Thomas R. Russell

> This article examines the state of the medical and surgical
> workforce, and how business-based and economic principles
> such as supply and demand have continued to shape it.
> Specifically, this article focuses on the following topics: past and
> present efforts to determine physician supply; where workforce
> shortages are most apparent at this time; and the factors that are
> contributing to the current shortfalls and their broader implica-
> tions. In addition, the author looks ahead to determine what
> changes we need to support, promote, and make to meet our
> patients' evolving needs and expectations.

Graduate Medical Education in Surgery in the United States 811
Richard H. Bell, Melissa B. Banker, Robert S. Rhodes,
Thomas W. Biester, and Frank R. Lewis

> Each year, approximately 1000 graduating medical students enter
> 5-year residency programs in general surgery. Their salaries are
> funded by the federal government. Following 5 years of general
> surgery training, approximately 70% of graduates enroll in a
> specialty fellowship. Surgery training currently faces a number of
> challenges, including the diminishing attractiveness of surgery as a
> career, attrition from residency programs, mandated work hour
> limits, extensive service requirements in the hospital environment,

increasing specialization, and changing patient expectations about the role of residents in their care, among others. In the face of these challenges, the profession is beginning to respond to the need for positive change in the process of training surgeons.

Certification and Maintenance of Certification in Surgery 825
Robert S. Rhodes and Thomas W. Biester

The processes that lead to certification by the American Board of Surgery (ABS) emphasize surgeons' training and qualifications. Moreover, the need for periodic recertification appears to provide strong motivation for surgeons to remain current. Such certification is regarded as having great value among patients, but concerns about quality and safety have increased pressure to assess what surgeons actually do in practice. As a result, the American Board of Medical Specialties (ABMS) member boards have recently initiated Maintenance of Certification (MOC) programs that add a requirement for assessment of practice performance to the elements of traditional certification. This article describes the current ABS certification process and the ABS MOC program in greater detail.

Assessing the Quality of Surgical Care 837
Aaron S. Fink, Kamal M. Itani, and Darrell C. Campbell, Jr

Because of better educated patients, more demanding payers, and regulatory agencies, safety and quality have become prominent criteria for evaluating surgical care. Providers are increasingly asked to document these areas, and patients are using this documentation to select surgeons and hospitals. Payers are using the data to direct patients to providers, and potentially to adjust reimbursement rates. Therefore, health care policy makers, health service researchers, and others are aggressively developing and implementing quality indicators for surgical practice. Given the complex interplay of structure, process, and outcomes, assessment of surgical quality presents a daunting task. We must firmly establish the links between these elements to validate current and future metrics, while engendering "buy-in" on the part of surgeons.

Safe Introduction of New Procedures and Emerging Technologies in Surgery: Education, Credentialing, and Privileging 853
Ajit K. Sachdeva and Thomas R. Russell

Ongoing horizon scanning is needed to identify new procedures and emerging technologies that should be evaluated for introduction into surgical practice. Following evidence-based evaluation, if a new modality is found ready for adoption in practice, surgeons need education in the safe and effective use of the new modality. The educational experience should include structured teaching and learning, verification of new knowledge and skills, preceptoring or proctoring, and monitoring of outcomes. Credentialing and privileging to perform a new procedure or use an emerging technology should be based on evaluation of knowledge and skills and outcomes of surgical care, and not merely on the numbers of procedures performed. Education of the surgical team is also essential. The entire process involving education, verification of knowledge and skills, credentialing, and privileging must be transparent. Patients need to play a central role in making informed decisions regarding their care that involves use of a new procedure or an emerging technology, and they should participate actively in their perioperative care.

Patient Safety and Quality in Surgery 867
Michael H. McCafferty and Hiram C. Polk

Patient safety and quality of care are inextricably linked. Surgery encompasses such a wide spectrum of diagnosis, treatment, postoperative care, and outpatient follow-up of so many illnesses that quality improvement and patient safety opportunities are numerous and potentially overwhelming. The study of error can be applied across all components of the care process, and offers many points of study to improve patient safety. A fundamental premise is that appropriate and safely delivered health care is less expensive. In our current climate, this emphasis on quality and safety will remain a high priority. Surgeon leadership at all levels is key to our professional viability.

Employers Flex Their Muscles as Health Care Purchasers 883
Suzanne Delbanco

Engaged health care purchasers–both individual and group–can stimulate some good, healthy competition in the health care system, and competition needs to be based on results. To determine results, we need accepted measures of quality and efficiency that make sense. Then, performance on those measures must be disclosed publicly. Only when this information is available to consumers and other purchasers of health care will they be able to make informed choices and reward effective and efficient health care providers.

The Role of the Expert Witness 889
Laurance Jerrold

The role of expert witnesses in medical malpractice litigation is often misunderstood. Much maligned, the expert has been the subject of castigation by a range of people, from his professional colleagues to the jurists who preside over his testimony. From an academic perspective, the expert witness is a necessary evil, and his denigration is his own doing; for the expert is a neutral character who creates his own professional persona. This purpose of this article is to serve as a primer for those interested in understanding the role that the expert is supposed to play in litigation, and the factors surrounding his activities.

A Comprehensive Primer of Surgical Informed Consent   903
James W. Jones, Lawrence B. McCullough, and Bruce W. Richman

Informed consent plays a major role in forming a therapeutic alliance with the patient. The informed consent process has evolved from simple consent, in which the surgeon needed only to obtain the patient's permission for a procedure, into informed consent, in which the surgeon provides the patient with information about clinically salient features of a procedure, the patient understands this information adequately, and the patient voluntarily authorizes the surgeon to perform the procedure. Special circumstances of informed consent include conflicting professional opinions, consent with multiple physicians, patients who are undecided or refuse surgery, patients with diminished decision-making capacity, surrogate decision making, pediatric assent, and consent for the involvement of trainees.

Withdrawing Life-Sustaining Treatment: Ethical Considerations   919
Sharon Reynolds, Andrew B. Cooper, and Martin McKneally

Withdrawing life-supporting technology from patients who are irremediably ill is morally troubling for caregivers, patients, and families. Interventions that enable clinicians to delay death create situations in which the dignity and comfort of dying patients may be sacrificed to spare professionals and families from their elemental fear of death. Understanding of the limits of treatment, expertise in palliation of symptoms, skillful communication, and careful orchestration of controllable events can help to manage the withdrawal of life support appropriately.

The Effect of Patients' Noncompliance on Their Surgeons' Obligations   937
Jay A. Jacobson

Effective physicians recognize that most patients have difficulty following instructions for a variety of reasons. That difficulty is best understood as nonadherence rather than noncompliance. The surgeon's role is to make the patient's choice informed, to be aware of the risk factors for nonadherence, and not to make adherence any more difficult than it has to be. The patient's role is to make choices between value-laden alternatives. Society's role is to distribute scarce medical resources equitably to patients who can and want to adhere to the necessary regimen to benefit from them.

The Global Impact of Surgical Volunteerism   **949**

Kathleen M. Casey

The significance of volunteer surgical outreach extends beyond the results achieved between individual physician and patient. Thus importance of the clinical, societal, political, educational, and economic impact of volunteerism is becoming better understood. This article examines the breadth and significance of such efforts.

Index   **961**

FORTHCOMING ISSUES

October 2007
Vascular Surgery
Benjamin Starnes, MD, *Guest Editor*

December 2007
Benign Disorders of the Pancreas
Stephen Behrman, MD, *Guest Editor*

RECENT ISSUES

June 2007
Inflammatory Bowel Disease
Joseph J. Cullen, MD, *Guest Editor*

April 2007
Breast Cancer
Lisa A. Newman, MD, MPH, *Guest Editor*

February 2007
Trauma
Ronald V. Maier, MD, *Guest Editor*

December 2006
Critical Care for the General Surgeon
Juan Carlos Puyana, MD
and Matthew R. Rosengart, MD, MPH *Guest Editors*

October 2006
Topics in Organ Transplantation for General Surgeons
Paul Morrissey, MD, *Guest Editor*

August 2006
**Recent Advances in the Management of Benign
and Malignant Colorectal Diseases**
Robin P. Boushey, MD, PhD
and Patricia L. Roberts, MD, *Guest Editors*

June 2006
Surgical Response to Disaster
Robert M. Rush, Jr, MD, *Guest Editor*

ELSEVIER
SAUNDERS

Surg Clin N Am 87 (2007) xi–xiv

SURGICAL
CLINICS OF
NORTH AMERICA

Foreword

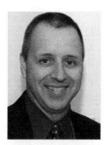

Ronald F. Martin, MD
Consulting Editor

A state of confusion is a good place from which to start. Recognizing that one is confused about something is somewhat essential to becoming uncon-fused. The problem with confusion, however, is that sometimes everybody is confused and sometimes one is alone is his confusion—the latter of which is merely reflective of lacking education or poor analytical capabilities. The genesis of this issue stems out of my trying to ascertain whether my igno-rance about certain aspects of our profession was unique to me, or was the confusion that I possessed more widespread. I have had the luxury of talking directly with many of our profession's leaders over the past couple of decades, and they have really tried to improve my understanding of how surgery and surgeons fit into society. Despite the very kind attentive-ness that has been afforded me by some extremely wise and busy people, I am still confused. Part of the reason for that is undoubtedly due to my own intellectual challenges, but part of it most certainly arises from the fact that as surgeons, we have collectively made little attempt to truly define our role in society in concrete terms. Without doubt, we have a substantial his-tory of how we view ourselves in lofty terms and vague attributes—we would all agree that we should be compassionate, caring, and technically proficient and put the needs of our patients ahead of our own. But those attributes are a bit hard to quantify and therefore easy to claim without hav-ing to prove.

One approach to dealing with "overwhelming" problems is to break them down into collections of problems that are surmountable and proceed to deal with them by bits. Assuming that each problem is manageable and that

0039-6109/07/$ - see front matter © 2007 Elsevier Inc. All rights reserved.
doi:10.1016/j.suc.2007.07.019
surgical.theclinics.com

there is enough time, one can usually solve the original question by some means. Some aspects of this issue are examples of my personal failure, to some degree, to address these assumptions: manageable problems and time.

The original proposition for this issue was made almost a decade ago, many years before I was asked to be the Consulting Editor for this series. The topic was viewed as interesting, but we did not know where to fit it into the series at that time; thus we wrote an issue on cancer instead. We were pretty sure that most surgeons would feel that cancer treatment was something a surgeon should know about. Several years later, a number of changes started to occur; the federal desire to train fewer specialists and more generalists gained traction, the 80-hour work week was imposed for residency training, the American Board of Surgery introduced the Maintenance of Certification concept, and the Residency Review Committee introduced its core competencies to name but a few changes. It was becoming clearer and clearer that the landscape for training and employing surgeons was shifting under our feet. As such, the proposal for this issue was resurrected with the intent of looking at the topics that influence our role as surgeons in medical systems and society in a single collection of reviews.

We decided to break the issue into components. The first set of topics would address the following issues: from where to recruit surgeons, and how many and of what type are needed; how to train them and decide that they are competent; and how to evaluate their continued education and training as well as certify it. The next set of topics was designed to address how surgeons fit into organizations and how to measure not just individual performance but performance within a system, as well as how performance data are released and for what purpose should they be used. The last set of topics was perhaps the most unusual. In this group, we offered an opportunity for representatives from different segments of society to tell us what they want or need from us. Examples of groups that were solicited include major industrial corporations that have been besieged by increasing financial burdens for health care, political figures seeking election at the presidential level who have espoused their desire for a change in the health care system, consumer advocacy groups, and economic advisers to government.

The Leapfrog Group responded to our request as you will read. As much as I would dearly love to name those who did not respond (especially those seeking your vote), it would probably be unwise. Suffice it to say that not a single response, even to say "No, thanks," was garnered from any individual seeking elected office or from any political party organization to voice an individual or collective opinion about how they feel that we as physicians or surgeons could better serve the needs of their constituencies. As for the corporations, each that was offered was, in fact, kind enough to reply that they were not interested.

Of further interest to me was that every single physician I approached either agreed to contribute or put me in touch with someone who could contribute in the event that his or her schedule was too tight. One can make of this what one will, but I personally find it interesting that considering the degree of complaint about our industry, the only people who people willing to suggest solutions were the ones being criticized. The Leapfrog group remains a notable exception.

I mentioned earlier that this issue was an example of failure of two kinds: manageable problems and time. In this instance, they are both personal failures of mine. This issue will most likely arrive to its subscribers late. It will not be through fault of the contributors nor the publishers nor my co-editor, Dr Vijay Khatri, but because of my delays. By way of explanation, and by no means an excuse, when we began this issue we were already on a tight schedule to work around some other unexpected occurrences. Shortly thereafter, I found myself unexpectedly back in Iraq, where we became somewhat preoccupied with local events. Despite best efforts, communication was slow and not always as reliable as one may have wished for. To whatever degree that it may have hampered others' ability to contribute to this issue, I am solely responsible. In particular, I owe an apology to Dr. Andrew Warshaw. Dr. Warshaw was quite willing to contribute a section on the roles of surgeon as political activists. Because of a loss of materials sent between him and me, we became incapable of meeting his scheduling needs. I assure you and Dr. Warshaw that should he wish, we will find a way to incorporate his information into a future issue.

As to the issue of a "manageable problem," I feel that I may have failed a bit there as well. It has been my assumption that a resolution to the perceived problems was in many respects desirable. After navigating this process, however, I have developed a skepticism (founded or otherwise) that this may not be the case. The business that we surgeons participate in is an enormous economic enterprise. Any real solution to our problems will involve significant change, and change will have profound economic implications for many—some good, some bad. There is much to be gained by many to keep the problem vocal and visible yet unresolved. In my opinion, there will be no ideal solution to our difficulties—if there were, we would have enacted it a long time ago. If the willing cast of participants in this issue are indicative of the individuals to whom we can turn for cooperation, I would suggest that we cannot wait for government or industry to address the big topics—it could be a while.

It seems to be an imperative for us to continue to study our needs and the needs of our patients. We must be careful not to confuse necessity with desire. Clearly, we shall be asked—directly or indirectly—to do more with less, and it will be upon us to figure out how to make that happen. Our patients, wittingly or otherwise, are counting on us to help improve this complicated system. Furthermore, because everybody is "pre-op," including us, there is an element of self-preservation both professionally and personally in our developing workable solutions.

As always, comment from the readership of this series is desired and welcome. I am sure these topics will persist. Any ideas about how we can address these concerns better or differently are solicited. Who knows—perhaps one of you will be asked to compile your own collection of ideas for future publication.

I again would like to thank those who have been so supportive in this project despite the extreme obstacles that were placed in our way. Our publishers at Elsevier, in particular our executive publisher, Catherine Bewick, have been kind above and beyond the call of duty in their tolerance of shifting timetables with this issue. I would also like to very personally thank the members of Task Force 3ʳᵈ Medical Command, Task Force 28ᵗʰ Combat Support Hospital (forward) and Task Force 399ᵗʰ Combat Support Hospital (forward), with special thanks to COL Leroy Winfield, COL Frederick Palmquist, COL Gregory Quick, LTC Wayne Mosley, and COL Patrick J. Sullivan, without whose professional and personal support during challenging times this issue would have been aborted. Their sacrifices and actions for our country and those injured in Iraq cannot be acknowledged enough.

Ronald F. Martin, MD
Department of Surgery
Marshfield Clinic
1000 North Oak Avenue
Marshfield, WI 54449, USA

E-mail address: martin.ronald@marshfieldclinic.org

ELSEVIER
SAUNDERS

Surg Clin N Am 87 (2007) xv–xvi

SURGICAL
CLINICS OF
NORTH AMERICA

Preface

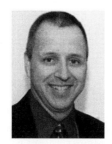 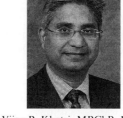

Ronald F. Martin, MD   Vijay P. Khatri, MBChB, FACS
Guest Editors

> No enterprise can exist for itself alone. It ministers to some great need, it performs some great service, not for itself, but for others; or failing therein, it ceases to be profitable and ceases to exist.
>
> —Calvin Coolidge

The intent of this issue of the *Surgical Clinics of North America* is to try to examine the role that our profession of surgery plays within a broader social context. It has become apparent to even the most casual observer over the past two decades that the topics of clinical relevance that used to dominate our conversations have been largely replaced with topics such as reimbursement, regulation, and our interactions with insurance companies, government, and the legal system. The national political agenda was virtually focused on health care reform and even credited with being the sole determinant of some elections until terrorism and the recent military conflicts essentially blotted out the sun on such debates. Through these changes, physicians and surgeons have had to try to sort out what in addition to being good doctors we have to do to serve our constituency—the patients.

We have reached out to contributors for this issue who will help to illuminate on various related issues; how we acquire and develop the work force, how we will address assessing and securing quality performance, maintenance of certification, and how we will interact with government and the legal system. We acknowledge that there are many topics that we have not covered or have not covered as fully as we could have or would have liked. This issue, like all the others in this series, is designed to review topics and act as a synopsis of thought-provoking information and a spring-board for further inquiry by the interested reader. By being involved as strong advocates for our own profession, we will secure the future we seek.

We would like to acknowledge with great appreciation those who contributed to this issue. Each person who undertook this effort has had to incorporate this task into an already overflowing schedule. In most respects, these contributors exemplify the rule that if you need something important done, turn to the person who is most busy and has the least time to deliver.

We would also very much like to express our deepest appreciation to Catherine Bewick, our executive publisher. Her unwavering patience and tireless support have allowed this issue to come together as it is despite over-whelming obstacles. We cannot thank her enough.

It is our hope that this issue will unravel some of the mysteries of the sometimes seemingly random business of surgery and will inspire the reader to learn more and engage in being a surgeon and a leader at any level. As surgeons we must all be willing, first and foremost, to put patient and work-place safety at the top of the priority list, while maintaining the integrity and ethical values of our discipline. We are deeply in need of engaging in determining our destiny for the sake of ourselves and more importantly for those whom we serve.

Ronald F. Martin, MD
Department of Surgery
Marshfield Clinic
1000 North Oak Avenue
Marshfield, WI 54449, USA

E-mail address: martin.ronald@marshfieldclinic.org

Vijay P. Khatri, MBChB, FACS
Professor of Surgery
Division of Surgical Oncology
University of California, Davis Cancer Center
4501 X Street, Sacramento, CA 95817, USA

E-mail address: vijay.khatri@ucdmc.ucdavis.edu

ELSEVIER
SAUNDERS

SURGICAL
CLINICS OF
NORTH AMERICA

Surg Clin N Am 87 (2007) 797–809

The Surgical Workforce: Averting a Patient Access Crisis

Thomas R. Russell, MD, FACS

American College of Surgeons, 633 N. Saint Clair Street, Chicago,
IL 60611-3211, USA

One of the critical questions affecting the future of our nation's health care system is whether we will have enough appropriately trained physicians—particularly surgical specialists—to meet the changing demands of American patients. Until recently, medical workforce studies typically forecast a surplus of specialists and a shortage of primary care physicians. Organized medicine, health policymakers, and representatives of medical education programs responded to these predictions by developing edicts aimed at fostering the production of generalists and constraining the growth of specialists.

Today, experts foresee a completely different scenario playing out—one in which patients will have difficulty accessing the surgical and other specialty services they will need. Our nation's emergency and rural health care centers are experiencing the most pervasive effects right now, although spot shortages are occurring elsewhere as well.

This article examines the state of the medical and surgical workforce, and how business-based and economic principles such as supply and demand have continued to shape it. Specifically, this article focuses on the following topics: past and present efforts to determine physician supply; where workforce shortages are most apparent at this time; and the factors that are contributing to the current shortfalls and their broader implications. In addition, the author looks ahead to determine what changes we need to support, promote, and make to meet our patients' evolving needs and expectations.

Determining physician supply and demand

Throughout the last century, policy experts sought to apply some sort of philosophical or economic theory to determine the number and types of

E-mail address: trussell@facs.org

health care professionals necessary to care for American patients. Some individuals point to the 1910 Flexner report as the nation's first foray into determining physician supply, because it implied that the United States was producing too many poorly trained physicians [1]. As a result of the Flexner report, medical schools that were educationally deficient were rightfully closed, and medical educators concentrated on creating "fewer but better doctors" [2].

After World War II, however, the demand for physicians grew in response to a number of societal shifts, including greater public affluence, an increasing number of college graduates, and pressure from the nation's underserved rural and inner-city areas [1]. Hence, in 1959 the Surgeon General's Consultant Group on Medical Education predicted a shortage of approximately 40,000 physicians in the United States by 1975. To prevent this situation from arising, President John F. Kennedy signed the Health Professions Education Assistance Act (P.L. 88-129) in 1963, stimulating the growth and expansion of US medical schools through the end of the 1970s. Between 1965 and 1980, the number of medical schools increased more than 69%, and the number of graduates went from 7409 to 15,135 annually [1].

Leading the nation's next major venture into assessing physician supply and demand was the Graduate Medical Education National Advisory Committee (GMENAC), which reported to the federal government. In 1981, GMENAC reported that the United States would have a surplus of 145,000 physicians by the year 2000. The report called for restricting the number of slots in medical schools as well as the number of international medical school graduates admitted into the country.

Soon thereafter, Congress created the Council on Graduate Medical Education (COGME), which concluded that the nation would experience a surplus of approximately 80,000 physicians by the year 2000, and predicted excessive growth in the specialties, including surgery. To constrain growth in the number of physicians, and particularly specialists, produced, COGME recommended that 50% of the new physicians enter generalist disciplines and 50% enter specialties. COGME also recommended limiting the number of residency training positions to 110% of the number of graduates of US medical schools, thereby stemming the influx of international medical graduates [3]. This policy became known as the 110/50/50 rule, and was the conventional wisdom for surgical education policies for the rest of the 20th century.

Paving the way for the policies of the 1990s was the Bureau of Health Professions in the Department of Health and Human Services, which reported to Congress that by 2000, the oversupply of physicians would reach 73,000. Meanwhile, various experts predicted that the managed care revolution of the 1990s would lessen the need for physicians. Hence, the Balanced Budget Act of 1997 (P.L. 105-33) capped the number of residency slots qualified for federal funding.

New approaches defy conventional wisdom

New methods of calculating physician supply and demand indicate that the restraints we have imposed on the production of medical and surgical professionals will lead to shortfalls in physician supply in the future. For example, R.A. Cooper [4], former dean of the Medical College of Wisconsin, posits that the demand for physicians parallels both economic and population growth. Cooper and his colleagues maintain that this correlation reflects underlying causal links between the nation's financial growth, its demand for care, and the consequent expectations for health care professionals to deliver services. Furthermore, Cooper and company note a pronounced connection between income and demand for specialty care. Thus, they project that as earnings ascend, the need for specialists will rise faster than the demand for generalists. This hypothesis contradicts the conventional wisdom that it is specialty growth that must be constrained [1].

A study published in 2003 [5] used a different approach to forecast surgical supply and demand. It combined age-specific rates of surgical procedures and their corresponding Medicare fee schedule relative value units to quantify the amount of surgical work that an average individual in a particular age group demands. Working from the assumption that age-specific, per capita use of surgical services will remain constant, the study authors project a 14% to 47% increase in the demand for all surgical services. The study concludes that because the American population is aging, the demand for surgical services will intensify [5]. In an editorial response, Jonasson [6] highlighted a deficiency in that study, noting that it predicted needs based on "established patterns of surgical use" and failed to account for the changing needs of patients. As Dr. Jonasson suggested, predictions pertaining to the need for surgical services are tenuous at best. Unquestionably, the American population is growing older, but it is difficult to estimate what types of care the next generation of seniors will require and expect to receive, given changes in attitude, financial security, and health concerns.

Other experts, such as Sheldon [7], of the University of North Carolina School of Medicine, say that all of the previously mentioned elements must be weighed in the physician supply and demand equation. More specifically, Sheldon maintains that age distribution and the economy are both important determinants of workforce needs, adding that a prosperous "graying" population will invest in health care and research.

Medical education policy advisers have only recently accepted these new approaches to measuring physician supply and demand, and now acknowledge that the United States is headed toward a physician shortage. Indeed, it was just in 2005 that the Association of American Medical Colleges and COGME agreed that physician shortfalls are likely to occur by 2020 [8]. Recent analyses undertaken for COGME by Edward Salsberg of the State University of New York at Albany estimate that shortage at 85,000 physicians [1]. Using this prediction and other assessments, COGME now forecasts that if the nation's population continues to use health care services as it has in the past, then a shortage of physicians is likely in the coming years. Moreover, COGME estimates that when supply and need for the coming years are calculated, the United States is projected to face a shortage of about 96,000 physicians in 2020 [9].

First signs of a workforce crisis

Symptoms of the burgeoning workforce shortage are already evident in facilities that provide care to some of the nation's most vulnerable populations—our trauma centers, emergency departments (EDs), and rural health facilities.

In June 2006, the Institute of Medicine (IOM) released a series of reports indicating that, "[A] national crisis in emergency care has been brewing and is now beginning to come into full view" [10]. The three reports—*Hospital-Based Emergency Care: at the Breaking Point; Emergency Medical Services: at the Crossroads*; and *Emergency Care for Children: Growing Pains*—identify what the IOM maintains are the most relevant issues facing the nation's emergency care system. Key problems highlighted in the reports include overcrowding, fragmentation, lack of disaster preparedness, shortcomings in pediatric emergency care, and, most relevant to this discussion, a shortage of specialists who will take emergency call [10].

The American College of Surgeons (ACS) points to similar trends in a "white paper" released in June 2006, titled *A Growing Crisis in Patient Access to Emergency Surgical Care* [11]. Based on data available from the American College of Emergency Physicians, the College found that nearly three quarters of ED medical directors believe they have inadequate on-call specialist coverage [12]. A study conducted by the Washington, DC,-based Lewin Group on behalf of the American Hospital Association showed that neurosurgeons, orthopedic surgeons, general surgeons, and plastic surgeons are among the specialists in short supply for ED on-call panels [13].

The inadequate number of specialists providing emergency call services is taking its toll on quality of care. In a recent survey, ED administrators acknowledged that the dearth of specialty coverage in the EDs poses a significant risk to patients. Furthermore, of those who indicated that they would avoid receiving care at their own ED (12%), 74% cited the lack of specialty reinforcement available [14].

Unfortunately, policymakers and researchers have given scant attention to the emergency workforce of the future, so more solid data are not yet available. Based on the information at hand, needless to say, the ACS concurs with the IOM's assertion that a growing shortage of surgical specialists available to cover our nation's EDs threatens prompt patient access to acute care services. As an organization that has long sought to improve the quality of trauma and emergency care through the standard-setting and educational programs conducted by our Committee on Trauma, the ACS is deeply concerned about the burgeoning emergency workforce shortage. Hence, we have been collaborating with the surgical specialty societies and with the IOM to determine why specialists decline to take emergency call, and to develop initiatives that will rectify this growing crisis.

Other sites that are experiencing the effects of the workforce losses are rural medical centers. The ACS Subcommittee on Rural Surgery has found that towns with fewer than 50,000 residents represent approximately 25% of the American population, but only 9% to 12% of the entire surgical workforce practices in nonmetropolitan areas. The absence of surgeons in rural areas leaves those individuals who do choose to practice outside of metropolitan locations in the position of having to spend more nights on call, often without assistance from appropriate specialists [15].

A canary in the coal mine

The problems that our nation's EDs, trauma centers, and rural hospitals are experiencing in and of themselves are causes for alarm and require immediate responses. Even more disturbing, however, is the likelihood that these situations represent what some of my colleagues refer to as "a canary in the coal mine." That is to say, if we fail to address the roots of these issues immediately, even more patients will experience diminished access to specialty care.

Our analysis of the emergency workforce crisis indicates that three broad yet tightly intertwined factors are contributing to the decreasing supply of surgeons: reimbursement, liability, and declining interest in critical specialties with movement toward subspecialization.

Arguably, the single greatest deterrent to pursuing a surgical career and to providing emergency services once in practice is declining reimbursement. The fact of the matter is that a significant proportion of emergency services are uncompensated. A report issued by the Center for Studying Health System Change indicates that surgical specialists are more likely than other specialists or primary care physicians to provide charitable care, probably because of the on-call mandates at their hospitals [16]. Meanwhile, payments from Medicare and Medicaid have been dropping, and insurance payments for elective procedures have decreased steadily over the past 2 decades because many private insurers model their payment policies on the Medicare fee schedule [11].

All physicians have concerns about the Medicare payment system, particularly its reliance on the sustainable growth rate (SGR) to calculate the conversion factor; however, its flaws are especially problematic for surgical specialists. Medicare services generally are growing a rate that allows many physicians to offset per-service payment reductions by increasing the volume of services they provide. Surgeons are unable to take advantage of this approach because the volume of surgical procedures provided is shrinking. New technology and advances in medications are resulting in safer, less costly alternatives to open procedures, thereby making many operations obsolete. Hence, surgeons have no means of offsetting payment cuts other than working longer hours—an action that fewer surgeons, particularly younger ones, are willing to take. Disincentives to providing Medicare services are cause for rising concern, in that the baby boomers will start becoming eligible for benefits in just a few years.

As another means of averting financial difficulties, some surgeons stop performing risky or less profitable operations. For example, a recent survey of neurosurgeons revealed that 38% now limit the types of procedures they perform, typically eliminating pediatrics, trauma-related services, and cranial procedures from their practices. By keeping the number of high-risk operations they conduct to a minimum, surgeons are less likely to be exposed to liability lawsuits. Again, the effects of this trend are most notable in the nation's EDs. Part of physicians' growing reluctance to take call stems from genuine worries that ED patients will sue. Furthermore, some surgeons have concluded that they simply cannot afford the added liability risk for a largely uninsured patient population [11].

Furthermore, younger surgeons are leaving states with the most severe liability problems. For example, in July 2005 the Project on Medical Liability in Pennsylvania, funded by the Pew Charitable Trust, reported, "Resident physicians in high-risk fields such as general surgery and emergency medicine named malpractice costs as the reason for leaving the state three times more often than any other factor" [17]. Moreover, an American Hospital Association study showed that more than 50% of hospitals in medical liability crisis states, many of which have large rural populations, now have difficulty recruiting physicians [18].

As surgeons seek to maintain their incomes and decrease their liability exposure, fewer are entering the specialties that provide most of the critical care in this country, including general surgery and neurosurgery. The ACS has found that shortages exist across a range of medical disciplines, but are particularly significant for surgery. The workforce in nonsurgical specialties has grown steadily over time, whereas the number of individuals entering surgery each year has remained relatively stable for more than 2 decades [11]. One possible explanation for this situation is that past predictions about the medical and surgical workforce led training programs to cap the number of individuals they accept. For instance, approximately 130 neurosurgery residency spots are available each year. On the opposite end of the spectrum, more than 4700 internal medicine positions are offered annually [19]. Considering the small number of neurosurgeons practicing in the United States today (approximately 3200), the large percentage over age 55 (34%), and the length of neurosurgical training, it will be difficult to replace a shrinking pool of competent neurosurgeons participating in on-call panels [11].

Although the number of critical care surgical specialists is decreasing, we are witnessing a growing movement toward subspecialization. Some surgeons are seeking to minimize financial disruptions by subspecializing in narrow fields dominated by elective services, such as breast surgery. In some cases, surgeons who narrow their scope of practice are able to omit hospital-based care from their repertoire by performing all procedures at ambulatory centers or in other outpatient settings. Some of these surgical specialists have established their own specialty facilities (boutique centers) that are equipped to provide only a small range of nonemergency procedures. In any event, surgeons who operate outside of the hospital setting become unavailable for emergency on-call panels [11].

Program directors, professors of surgery, and other individuals familiar with resident matches report that at least 50% to 70% of general surgeons pursue fellowship training following categorical general surgery training. In addition, more institutions are offering fellowships that lack formal accreditation oversight, including minimally invasive fellowships, accelerating the phenomenon of early specialization [20]. As their scope of practice narrows, an alarming trend has emerged—many surgeons no longer feel qualified to manage the range of problems they are likely to encounter in an ED (Thomas R. Russell, MD, personal communication, 2006).

In addition to payment and liability, another possible motive for increased subspecialization is the lifestyle it affords. That is to say, younger surgeons may be inclined to narrow their practices to allow more time for raising families and pursuing outside interests. The implications of this trend are of concern, especially in light of the fact that surgeons are retiring earlier. For example, currently general surgeons are retiring around age 60. Previously, the typical retirement age for general surgeons was 72 [20].

Addressing immediate concerns

Because the problems we are seeing in urgent care centers and rural facilities are coming to full boil, it's safe to assume that many of these issues will soon spill over into the broader American population. Hence, our immediate concern must be lowering the flames burning beneath the surface of the emergency workforce crisis. Because so many of these problems relate to government policies, all stakeholders will need to collaborate in the development of socioeconomic solutions.

To encourage surgeons to take call in our nation's EDs and trauma centers, policymakers should revisit how they enforce the Emergency Medical Treatment and Active Labor Act (EMTALA). This 1986 law was enacted to curtail patient-dumping. Over the years, regulators have interpreted EMTALA in a highly restrictive sense, and imposed unbearable burdens on specialists who provide emergency coverage. Although the federal government has taken steps to address some of the law's most serious flaws, specialists continue to perceive EMTALA as a mandate to provide around-the-clock uncompensated care. The College intends to work with regulators to continue refining EMTALA and related legislation to encourage specialists to provide emergency care.

Additionally, we need to address reimbursement issues. To limit concerns about providing uncompensated care, the federal government needs to comprehensively address the increasing number of Americans without health insurance. Moreover, we need to replace the SGR with a more equitable means of determining Medicare payment. Presently, policymakers are taking steps to implement value-based purchasing, which would reward physicians and other providers who have better outcomes with higher payment levels. The ACS is working with federal legislators and the Center for Medicare and Medicaid Services (CMS) to ensure that any such methodology accounts for the unique nature of surgery.

To alleviate physicians' concerns about providing uncompensated care, the ACS suggests that the federal government provide some tax relief for these services. Furthermore, we believe Medicare should support those hospitals that pay stipends to physicians who take call.

With regard to improving access to care in rural areas, one action that the government could take is to expand the 5% bonus Medicare pays to individuals who practice in physician scarcity areas to include the range of locations where rural patients receive care. Under the current construct, bonus payments are based on site of service, making the program more appealing to primary care physicians who are likely to have offices in small towns. Rural surgeons tend to work either in regional hospitals or in offices near those institutions, which are often located in more populated areas. As a result, the site of surgical service may be outside a physician scarcity area.

In addition, National Health Service Corps scholarship and medical school loan repayment plans should be extended to all medical students who agree to complete a period of service in an underserved rural or inner-city location. Currently this program is unavailable to surgeons and other specialists.

The ACS plans to work with Congress to create a health professions support program to cover medical school debt for young surgeons who work in community or rural hospitals/trauma centers. We also will negotiate with policymakers to refine current laws pertaining to physician specialty shortage areas, so they may more effectively encourage surgical specialists to provide care in locations where the demand is greatest.

To alleviate medical liability concerns, the United States needs to enact comprehensive reforms. Until a legislative solution emerges, however, interim steps should be considered. For example, policymakers could limit exposure to litigation and provide qualified immunity for EMTALA care by bringing these mandated services under the Federal Tort Claims Act.

With respect to ensuring prompt access to surgical care for severely injured patients, the ACS continues to advocate for reauthorization of the Trauma Care Systems Planning and Development Act of 1990. Administered through the Health Resources and Services Administration, in the past several years this program has distributed $31.4 million in funds to all 50 states and five territories for the purpose of developing state and regional trauma care systems. But even with this influx of federal funds, only one fourth of the United States population lives in an area with a trauma center.

In addition, some experts are calling for the creation of acute care or emergency care surgeons. Surgeons trained in this new specialty would be trained in the range of procedures commonly performed by general surgeons on patients who have experienced a traumatic injury and critical surgical conditions, such as appendicitis. Typically, acute care surgeons would be salaried employees, rather then private practitioners struggling to balance their elective caseloads with emergency call, a concept that resonates with many young people. The surgical specialties have diverse opinions about the necessity of creating this new specialty, and the range of emergency and nonemergent services it would embrace, and the ACS is encouraging all sides to work together to determine how these individuals would be trained and the extent of their responsibilities.

Finally, it is vitally important that policy researchers and policymakers gain a greater understanding of the forces that are undermining our nation's emergency care system. Studies of the growing uninsured population, for example, should focus not only on access to care for chronic illnesses, but also on access to acute care services. The ACS is committed to initiating this dialog, and will continue to collaborate with representatives of all surgical specialties in order to improve our understanding of the problems confronting surgical practice today, and to develop innovative solutions to them.

Looking ahead: a macroscopic view

The steps just mentioned will address the nation's immediate concerns about providing physician services to emergency patients and underserved populations, and should have a spill-over effect on the workforce in general. More specifically, these initiatives are likely to make entering key specialties more attractive to young people who are concerned about payment, liability, and lifestyle issues. But what changes in the health care environment do we need to anticipate, and how do we address them now to secure a stable and appropriate workforce for the future?

In light of the likely gap between the expected supply, demand, and need for physicians in the future, COGME now recommends implementation of new strategies. For example, to meet the future physician workforce demand in the United States (particularly given the aging baby boom population), COGME recommends that the number of physicians entering residency training each year be increased from approximately 24,000 in 2002 to 27,000 in 2015. The council also suggests that the distribution of generalists and specialists reflect an ongoing assessment of demand for medical service. Hence, COGME no longer recommends a rigid national numerical target for the mix of specialists and generalists [9].

Other COGME recommendations include increasing total enrollment in United States medical schools by 15% from their 2002 levels over the next decade, and phasing in an increase in the number of residency and fellow-ship positions eligible for Medicare funding. COGME also calls for the development of systems to track the supply, demand, need for, and distribution of physicians, as well as comprehensive reassessment to guide future decisions about medical education capacity [9].

In addition, COGME asserts that additional specialty-specific studies are needed to better understand physician workforce needs, and to inform the medical education community and policymakers of the nation's specialty-specific needs. Furthermore, COGME suggests promoting increased physician productivity, through activities such as providing funding to evaluate alternative models of care and practice and organizational arrangements, evaluation of new technologies, dissemination of information to physicians about the efficacy of advancements in patient care, and introduction of reimbursement policies that support productivity enhancements. And, finally, COGME recommends that we expand programs and develop policies that address the geographic maldistribution of physicians, improve access to care for underserved populations and communities, promote appropriate specialty distribution and deployment, encourage workforce diversity, and support analyses of data related to these issues [9]. COGME's recommendations are certainly worth pursuing, because they respond to the fact that our concept of generalist versus specialist supply and demand is evolving, largely in light of changes in the medical marketplace.

The ACS intends to continue to monitor the evolution of specialties, the distribution of specialties by state and region, liability issues, and reimbursement issues, as well as their effects on patient access to care. We also anticipate that we will continue to collaborate with specialty societies to formulate policies that address the workforce situation and to develop data that tracks the dynamic workforce shifts occurring annually. Our goal is to encourage public policies rooted in ensuring that 21st century patients receive surgical services from an adequate number and appropriately trained mix of specialists.

Perhaps most importantly, we also need to take an unflinching look at how industrialization and advances in technology are redefining what it means to be a surgeon, a medical specialist, or even a generalist in the 21st century. We also need to consider how health system reforms are likely to affect patients' needs, and thereby alter our perception of what it means to be a surgeon or physician.

Cooper [4], for example, says that the medical professions are being forced to redefine themselves in ever more narrow scientific and technological spheres. In addition, he predicts that symptom control, treatment of minor and self-limited disorders, chronic disease management, primary care, and multisystem care will become the shared responsibility of both physicians and nonphysician clinicians. Consequently, physicians will be concentrated in the most specialized and technological areas of medicine, particularly complex and multisystem care.

Given the technological advances that have occurred within the last several decades, and encroachment from other disciplines, surgeons probably are going to become providers of more comprehensive yet more specialized care. Already the insertion of stents, catheters, balloons, and so on are the first line of treatment for many conditions. Frequently, it is only after these alternatives have been exhausted that an open surgical repair takes place.

The movement toward less invasive procedures will undoubtedly continue in an era when safety, effectiveness, and cost control are the yardsticks for measuring the value of care. Hence, surgeons no longer will be able to maintain practices in which all they do is operate. Instead, vascular surgeons will evolve into vascular specialists, breast surgeons into breast specialists, bariatric surgeons into metabolic specialists, and so on. In other words, in the future surgeons will be not only capable providers of operative services, but professionals who are able to treat the whole surgical patient. We will need to understand and cure the underlying diseases and conditions that force patients to seek out the skills of surgeons in the first place.

This trend most likely will continue as medical researchers delve further into the molecular and genetic origins of human disease systems. As a result, our emphasis will shift from curing and eradicating disease on a per-patient basis to preventing or inhibiting its development and acuity in entire populations [21].

As providers of more comprehensive care, very few specialists will function autonomously. Rather they will be core members of teams of highly trained health care professionals. Teams formed within mature health systems will likely deliver care in multidisciplinary centers, where physicians, surgeons, and allied health personnel will work together to provide comprehensive and consistent patient care. The professionals at these centers will receive integrated training and credentialing, and experience integrated quality controls to maintain the same high standards of care throughout.

Centers based on this model already exist at forward-thinking institutions such as the Mayo Clinic, and encapsulate the sort of innovations we need to transfuse into the entire health care system and bring life to the concept of providing patient-based care. With an emphasis on treating the whole patient who has specific health issues, these centers will serve to promote wellness, prevention, and control of chronic conditions.

Furthermore, these centers are appealing to third-party payers. Because all services are provided at one facility, it is possible to put all charges on one bill. This arrangement eliminates the time and expense associated with verifying and paying multiple claims.

Needless to say, future specialists in surgery-related care will require different training than we have provided to surgeons in the past. They will need to be acquainted with noninvasive radiological and imaging techniques. They will need to understand the genetic and molecular causes of illness. They will need to be able to interact with and effectively lead the other professionals on the patient care team and to compassionately communicate with patients.

The ACS is seeking to help surgeons adapt to these changes by offering educational programs designed to encourage their growth as well-rounded professionals. We are introducing more opportunities for them to attain hands-on experience in minimally and noninvasive procedures. Additionally, we are introducing them in the skills needed to lead health care teams and foster the physician-patient relationship.

Finally, resident training programs will need to move their focus toward providing an environment in which physicians can develop these new competencies, continue to comply with 80-hour workweek mandates, and adapt to the lifestyle concerns of young people today. Consequently, a truncated training model is likely to emerge. Under the new prototype, medical students and residents with ambitions of entering surgery-related specialties may, for example, opt for 3 years of general surgery and 3 years of specialty training, including a medical rotation to ensure that individuals are able to provide certain nonoperative services. This approach will enable surgical specialists to become immersed in their true avocations more quickly, thereby increasing the appeal of postgraduate training for young people anxious to get on with their lives. Moreover, it will allow training programs to focus more specifically on inculcating residents in the broad range of skills that surgical specialists will need to possess. The Resident and Associate Society of the ACS is examining the potential for development of truncated specialty training programs.

Summary

This article should have provided the reader with a background into the forces that have shaped the surgical workforce in the past, described our present concerns, offered some solutions to these problems, and given insights into how we can strengthen the workforce to meet the demands of the future. As we continue to discuss physician supply and demand in this century, we must bear in mind that we are just beginning to see policy makers shift their emphasis in redesigning the health care system away from cost controls alone and more toward value-based care. Most likely, this movement away from applying market-based principles to our health care system will have profound effects on what we need to do to maintain a strong medical workforce.

References

[1] Blumethal D. New steam from an old cauldron—the physician-supply debate. N Engl J Med 2004;350(17):1780–7.
[2] Ludmerer KM. Time to heal: American medical education from the turn of the century to the era of managed care. New York: Oxford University Press; 1999.
[3] Council on Graduate Medical Education. Summary of eighth report: patient care physician supply and requirements: testing COGME recommendations. Washington, DC: Council on Graduate Medical Education. Available at: http://www.cogme.gov/rpt8_3.htm. Accessed February 1, 2007.

[4] Cooper RA. Preparing for a future with too few physicians. The Mildred C.J. Pfeiffer Lecture at the College of Physicians of Philadelphia (PA), November 9, 2006.

[5] Etzoni DA, Liu JH, Maggard MA, et al. The aging population and its impact on the surgery workforce. Ann Surg 2003;238:170–7.

[6] Jonasson O. "I prefer old age to the alternative": Maurice Chevalier, 1962. Ann Surg 2003; 238:178–9.

[7] Sheldon GF. Great expectations: the 21st century health workforce. Am J Surg 2003;185: 35–41.

[8] Association of American Medical Colleges. Medical school expansion plans: results of the AAMC 2005 survey of U.S. medical schools. Center for Workforce Studies. Available at: http://www.aamc.org/meded/cfws/enroll.pdf. Accessed May 18, 2006.

[9] Council on Graduate Medical Education. Physician workforce policy guidelines for the United States, 2000-2020: 16th report. Available at: http://www.cogme.gov/report16.htm. Accessed February 1, 2007.

[10] Institute of Medicine Committee on the Future of Emergency Care in the United States Health System. Report brief. Washington, DC: National Academy of Science; 2006.

[11] Division of Advocacy and Health Policy, American College of Surgeons. A growing crisis in patient access to emergency surgical care. Bull Am Coll Surg 2006;91(8):8–19.

[12] American College of Emergency Surgeons. On-call specialist coverage in U.S. emergency departments, American College of Emergency Physicians Survey of Emergency Department Directors. Available at: http://www.acep.org/NR/rdonlyres/DF81A858-FD39–46F6-B46A-15DF99A45806/0/RWJ_OncallReport2006.pdf. Accessed May, 2006.

[13] The Lewin Group analysis of AHA ED hospital capacity survey, 2002. April 2002, 7–18. Available at: http://www.aha.org/ahapolicyforum/resources/Eddiversionsurvey0404.html. Accessed April 4, 2006.

[14] The Schumacher Group. 2005 hospital emergency department administration survey. Available at: http://www.tsged.com/Survey2005.pdf. Accessed June, 2006.

[15] Hughes TG. Rural surgical practice: a personal perspective. Bull Am Coll Surg 2007;92(2): 12–7.

[16] Cunningham PJ, May JH. A growing hole in the safety net: physician charity care declines again. Tracking report 13. Center for Studying Health System Change. Available at: http://www.hschange.org/CONTENT/826/. Accessed March, 2006.

[17] The Project on Medical Liability in Pennsylvania. Available at: http://medliabilitypa.org/news/index.pjp?NewsID=15. Accessed June, 2006.

[18] American Hospital Association. American hospital association survey: professional liability insurance: a growing crisis (white paper). Washington, DC: AHA; 2003.

[19] Association of American Medical Schools. The National Residency Matching Program. Available at: http://www.nrmp.org/2006advdata.pdf. Accessed April 4, 2006.

[20] Sheldon GF. Workforce issues in general surgery. Am Surg 2007;73:100–8.

[21] von Eschenbach AC. The molecular metamorphosis: health care in the 21st century. Chicago: American Urological Association Lecture, 2006 Clinical Congress of the American College of Surgeons; 2006.

ELSEVIER
SAUNDERS

SURGICAL
CLINICS OF
NORTH AMERICA

Surg Clin N Am 87 (2007) 811–823

Graduate Medical Education in Surgery in the United States

Richard H. Bell, Jr, MD*, Melissa B. Banker, BA,
Robert S. Rhodes, MD, Thomas W. Biester, MS,
Frank R. Lewis, MD

*American Board of Surgery, 1617 John F. Kennedy Boulevard, Suite 860,
Philadelphia, PA 19103-1847, USA*

Graduate medical education in surgery currently consists of 5 or more years of post-medical school training. This training occurs in hospital-based residency programs, and is financed largely by the federal government. The traditional model of hospital-based surgical residency, in which aspiring surgeons participate in the care of patients under the tutelage of fully-trained surgeons, is a century old, and is under increasing scrutiny from patients, educators, and regulatory bodies. As the profession responds to these challenges, our current model of training may be on the brink of significant change.

Brief history of graduate medical education in surgery in the United States

The concept of the hospital-based residency in surgery is attributed to William S. Halsted, MD, [1] professor of surgery at Johns Hopkins University, who in 1904 advocated for a "system which will produce ... surgeons of the highest type." In the Halstedian model, several house officers began the Hopkins residency program each year, but half were only permitted to train for 1 year, and few completed a full course of training. This "pyramidal" style of residency was subsequently adopted by many hospitals. In the 1940s, Dr. Edward Churchill at the Massachusetts General Hospital proposed trading the "pyramidal" structure for a "rectangular" design in which all accepted residents were able to complete training [2], but the pyramidal nature of surgical training persisted at many programs until the 1980s, when

---

* Corresponding author.
E-mail address: rbell@absurgery.org (R.H. Bell, Jr).

the Residency Review Committee for Surgery (RRC) of the Accreditation Council on Graduate Medical Education (ACGME) began to require programs to choose the same number of starting residents as finishing residents. Such residents, guaranteed full training as long as their performance is satisfactory, are currently referred to as "categorical" residents. The number of categorical positions available in each general surgery residency is dictated by the RRC. In theory, the number of surgical training positions is also limited by the amount of federal funding to hospitals, but the RRC limit is the dominant factor in determining the number of surgical trainee positions available in the United States. Many hospitals would probably choose to fund additional resident positions out of their own revenues if the RRC limit were not in place. The RRC has been conservative about allowing new residency slots; as a result, the number of categorical positions in surgery has been relatively flat for the last 2 decades (Fig. 1).

In addition to categorical positions, residency programs are permitted to recruit "preliminary" residents, who are not guaranteed full 5-year training in general surgery. This group of residents is in turn divided into "designated" and "nondesignated" preliminary residents. Designated preliminary residents are those residents who have been offered full training in a specialty other than general surgery (for example, neurosurgery), but who complete 1 or more years of preparatory training in general surgery before entering their chosen specialty. In recent years, the number of designated preliminary positions in general surgery residencies has diminished as specialties such as orthopedic surgery and otolaryngology have chosen to take responsibility for the entire period of training of their residents.

Nondesignated preliminary residents are not offered full training in any surgical field, but are offered only a first-year residency position in general surgery. They may subsequently be offered a second year of preliminary status, but must be accepted into a categorical position after their second year

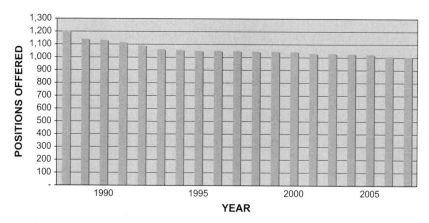

Fig. 1. The number of categorical R1 general surgery residency positions offered in the United States 1988-2006 (*Data courtesy of* National Resident Matching Program.)

to continue training. At the present time, residency programs are allowed to have a total number of nondesignated preliminary residents equal to twice the number of categorical entering positions. For example, a residency program that is allowed five categorical positions in its first-year residency class would be able to have at any given time a total of up to 10 nondesignated preliminary residents in the program.

Residency programs

There are currently 251 approved allopathic training programs in surgery in the United States. The programs vary in size; the average residency graduates 6 trainees per year, with the smallest graduating 1 trainee per year, and the largest approved to graduate 13. Of the 251 programs, approximately half are affiliated with medical schools, and the remainder are based in community hospitals not affiliated with a university. Altogether, these residency programs graduate approximately 1000 individuals each year. Of the 1000 graduates, about 300 go directly from residency into the practice of general surgery. The other 700 graduates enroll in additional training in cardiothoracic surgery, plastic surgery, vascular surgery, transplantation, advanced gastrointestinal surgery, surgical oncology, colorectal surgery, breast surgery, endocrine surgery, surgical critical care, or other subspecialties of general surgery.

In addition to the approximately 1000 people who graduate from allopathic training programs each year, about 80 osteopathic surgeons graduate annually from 30 US training programs.

Funding for graduate medical education in surgery

In 1966, as part of the landmark Medicare law, the federal government assumed the responsibility for funding graduate medical education (GME) in the United States. The Medicare-Medicaid program pays hospitals, not medical schools, for the training of residents. Medicare-Medicaid payments to hospitals for training in surgery currently amount to about 93% of the total budget for GME, with the remainder coming from the Department of Defense, Department of Veterans Affairs, and US Public Health Service. The current federal budget for GME is approximately $9 billion dollars per year, or approximately $90,000 dollars per resident per annum. Medicare funds for GME are dispersed to hospitals in two forms: direct medical education (DME) payments and indirect medical (IME) payments. DME payments are intended to provide direct salary support for residents and partial salary support for teachers, as well as to defray overhead costs of the educational program. Total annual DME payments to a hospital are based on a historical per-resident stipend, which is then multiplied by the number of residents in the hospital and multiplied by the fraction of total hospital in-patient days that are Medicare patient days. IME payments are also based upon the proportion of services provided by the hospital to Medicare beneficiaries. IME payment levels also depend upon the ratio of residents to hospital beds. IME funds are intended to compensate for the greater patient care expenses that teaching hospitals incur as a function of providing GME. The IME component of payment to hospitals is approximately twice the amount of the DME component. In 1997, the Balanced Budget Act enacted by the US Congress froze the level of resident positions paid for by Medicare, as well as the rates for some parts of the funding. There is currently debate about whether funding for GME should be provided by a different government mechanism, such as an endowment, or whether the federal government should be funding GME at all.

Resident salaries are determined by individual hospital programs, and typically range between $30,000 and $60,000 per year, rising with each year of training. In 2002, three former resident physicians filed a class-action antitrust lawsuit against the National Resident Matching Program (NRMP), which administers the senior medical student match program for residency positions, the ACGME, and 29 hospitals that sponsor residency programs, claiming that the match has restrained trade and kept salaries artificially low. The suit, Paul Jung, MD and colleagues vs. Association of American Medical Colleges, et al, was ultimately dismissed in 2004 after Congress intervened and passed legislation asserting that the NRMP process did not violate antitrust law.

Legal status of residents

Residents at publicly owned hospitals are considered government employees, and have been able to form unions since the 1957 National Labor Relations Act. In 2000, the National Labor Relations Board overturned its own long-standing policy and ruled that residents in private hospitals are also employees, giving all residents in the United States the right to form or join unions and engage in collective bargaining. Although all residents have had the ability to form collective bargaining units for the last 6 years, episodes of labor unrest at hospitals have been relatively rare.

Residents thus occupy the somewhat unusual position of being students and employees at the same time. No one disputes the necessity for learning during residency, but the legal status of residents as employees creates the potential for friction between hospitals, which can assert that residents have "service" responsibilities, and educators, who in general advocate for reducing service requirements and maximizing educational opportunities.

Regulatory oversight of graduate surgical education

The oversight of surgical GME in the United States falls largely to two organizations. The American Board of Surgery (ABS), founded in 1937 and located in Philadelphia, is responsible for assessing the knowledge of graduating residents, and certifies them based on an examination process. Candidates for ABS certification must be graduates of an ACGME approved residency program, and must pass the written (qualifying) examination of the ABS, a 300-item, multiple choice examination of cognitive knowledge, before being permitted to sit for the oral (certifying) examination, which is a 90-minute examination that assesses clinical judgment and decision-making.

The ABS takes the process of examination very seriously and conducts examinations in a scientific and professional manner. It has developed a question-writing training program for all of its examination committee members. Questions written for ABS examinations are scrutinized carefully in a multilevel review process and rewritten if necessary before they are used on an examination. The ABS employs a full-time psychometrician to evaluate the degree of difficulty and validity for all questions used on its written examinations.

Currently, approximately 20% of candidates taking the qualifying examination do not earn a passing grade on their first attempt. After having passed the qualifying examination, approximately 20% of candidates fail the oral (certifying) examination on their first attempt. Candidates are able to repeat either examination five times in 5 years. In the last decade, 5% to 6% of candidates could not pass the examinations on repeated attempts, and ultimately failed to become certified.

The ABS is an independent non-profit organization. Its directors (who review and select test items and administer the examinations) are volunteers. There are currently 31 ABS directors, all of whom are practicing surgeons. Twenty-eight are nominated by national academic and regional surgical societies, and there are three at-large directors. The ABS has a full-time executive director, two additional full-time physician staff members, a psychometrician, and several support personnel.

The ABS is one of 24 member boards of the American Board of Medical Specialties (ABMS), which encompasses all of the disciplines of allopathic medicine.

Because the ABS examines candidates for certification on the knowledge accumulated during residency, it in essence defines the educational content of surgical training. The ABS provides general guidelines as to the body of knowledge which it expects a certified surgeon to have mastered. These guidelines are modified as necessary as new knowledge enters the field of surgery and other knowledge becomes outdated.

In contrast to the ABS role of certifying individual surgeons, the RRC certifies that individual residencies are discharging their educational responsibilities successfully. The RRC is a unit of the ACGME, which is currently an independent corporation. It was founded in 1981 by the American Medical Association (AMA), the American Association of Medical Colleges (AAMC), the ABMS, the Council of Medical Specialty Societies (CMSS).

and the American Hospital Association (AHA). The ACGME is located in Chicago. It is charged with accrediting all medical core residency programs in the United States, and in addition accredits some, but not all, post-residency fellowships. In essence, the ABS is responsible for defining the body of knowledge required of trainees in surgery, whereas the RRC assures that individual residency programs provide the proper environment for residents to acquire the knowledge.

The program requirements of the RRC are rather detailed, and encompass areas such as the work environment, the curriculum, and the eligibility requirements for faculty and program directors. Professional ACGME inspectors review residency programs for compliance with RRC standards through an in-person site visit, and then report their findings to the RRC. Following a site-visit report, the RRC may grant a program full accreditation for a period of 5 years (the maximum) or less. Alternatively, it may grant conditional accreditation, and request that evidence be provided of satisfactory resolution of deficiencies. When more serious problems are present, the RRC may place a program on probationary status or revoke its accreditation. Currently, 95% of US residency programs are accredited, about half for the maximum period of 5 years; 2% are in the initial/provisional stage of accreditation, and 3% are in probationary or warning status.

The RRC has nine members, all of whom are surgeons. One member is a resident. The members are nominated for service by the American College of Surgeons (ACS), the ABS, and the AMA. In addition, the RRC has a full-time professional executive director and support staff.

Issues currently confronting graduate surgical education

Attractiveness of surgery as a career

For many years, more applicants from US medical schools applied for categorical surgical residency positions than the system could accept. In the 1990s, the number of applicants to surgical residency programs by US medical students began to fall. Between 1992 and 2002, the number of US medical school graduates who applied to general surgery residency programs fell from 1381 to 931, 100 less than the number of positions offered. In 2002, 7% of categorical residency positions went completely unfilled in the initial phase of the match. Since 2002, the trend has reversed, categorical positions are filling in the match, and increasing numbers of US students are applying for surgery programs, but not yet at historic levels (Fig. 2).

The decline in applications to surgery residency programs by US medical graduates has prompted a number of studies of medical student attitudes toward surgery as a career. Many of today's students view the lifestyle of a practicing surgeon as the primary deterrent to choosing surgery as a profession [3].

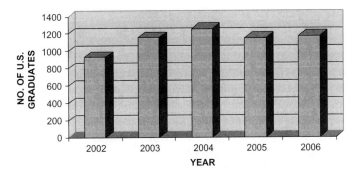

Fig. 2. The number of graduates of US medical schools applying for categorical general surgery training positions during the years 2002–2006. (*Data courtesy of* the National Resident Matching Program.)

There is a perception that surgery is not attractive to female medical students, who now constitute half of the student body in the US, but only one fourth of surgery residents. It is true that a smaller proportion of female medical students apply to surgery programs than their male counterparts, but an ABS study of residents in training reveal that the rate of increase in female residents has accelerated, and has been increasing by about 2% per year for the last 5 years, which will result in gender parity in surgery residency programs within the next 10 years (F. Lewis, unpublished data, 2006).

The question remains whether surgery is attracting top medical students. Data from the National Resident Matching Program (NRMP), which administers the residency match process, show that about 20% of students entering surgical residency programs are Alpha Omega Alpha honor society members. General surgery applicants are not on average as academically successful in medical school as those students entering other surgical specialties [4]. Students entering surgery residency are approximately equivalent to those entering internal medicine residency in terms of test scores and academic achievement. Of course, the generally high quality of US medical students guarantees that even average students are gifted, and it is not a given that surgery as a profession would be better served by attracting only the highest-achieving students.

In the meantime, the number of applicants to surgery residency programs from non-US medical schools has increased. By and large, international medical graduates (IMGs) fill surgical positions in residency programs that are not considered desirable by US medical school graduates. In 2006, 99 of 1046 categorical surgical positions (9.5%) were filled by IMGs. The success rate of US medical school graduates in the match for categorical positions is approximately 75% (3 out of 4 match to a position somewhere), whereas only one of 10 IMGs matches successfully to a categorical position. IMGs are more successful in obtaining nondesignated preliminary resident positions. Last year, 238 of 748 available preliminary positions were filled by IMGs.

Attrition from surgical residency programs

A major problem in surgical training is the attrition rate from categorical residency positions. RRC data [5] suggest that about 2% of all surgery residents are either terminated or withdraw from residency every year; however, their data use the total of categorical and preliminary residents as the denominator, and therefore may underestimate the losses from categorical training positions. Studies recently begun at the ABS suggest that the percentage of residents leaving categorical positions is much higher, and that approximately 20% or more of residents beginning a categorical surgery residency ultimately fail to complete it. Because the RRC has eliminated the "pyramid," filling vacant categorical positions usually involves moving a nondesignated preliminary resident into a categorical position, or accepting a resident in transfer from another program. Neither group represents a particularly optimal source for replacements—nondesignated preliminary residents are often those who failed to match to categorical positions in the first place, and transferring residents may have a history of underperformance. The data at ABS indicate that residents who train in more than two programs perform very poorly on our examinations.

Increasing subspecialization within general surgery

As knowledge has increased dramatically in surgery and as new technology has led to a steady expansion of the surgical therapeutic armamentarium, the broadly trained general surgeon capable of treating a wide variety of conditions in multiple organ systems has become a rarity. In the past 30 years, general surgery has calved a number of subspecialties, including relatively broad fields such as thoracic surgery, transplantation, oncology, and surgical critical care, as well as "niche" subspecialties such as breast surgery or bariatric surgery. Today's well-informed patients continue to drive the process of subspecialization by seeking out experts in particular diseases in lieu of a general surgeon. In addition, much has been written about the fact that practitioners who have significant experience with certain complex operations have better outcomes than surgeons who do the operation only occasionally [6], again reinforcing the value of a limited subspecialty practice.

Currently, 70% of the graduates of general surgery residencies opt for additional subspecialty training before entering practice. It is difficult to know with certainty all of the factors that are driving this sea change in surgical training. A great many residents, particularly those in large university-based programs, are exposed almost exclusively to subspecialists during their residency, and probably choose to emulate their mentors. Another factor undoubtedly driving the rapid growth in advanced surgical fellowships is the desire of faculty subspecialists to recruit motivated and experienced apprentices. Residents probably perceive competitive and financial advantages to subspecialization. Certain subspecialties also offer the likelihood of a more controllable lifestyle than traditional general surgery.

Unfortunately, the rapid proliferation of postresidency fellowships has created a self-fulfilling prophecy; as more and more operations are performed by postresidency fellows, residency training becomes less and less robust. As a result, many residents believe that general surgery training as it currently exists fails to prepare them adequately for practice, and so they feel compelled to seek additional training. Nowhere is this more apparent than in the extraordinary growth of postresidency fellowships in gastrointestinal surgery (now numbering well over 100), a field which has traditionally been at the core of general surgery.

It will be very difficult if not impossible to reverse the trend toward more and more subspecialization, but there are problems surfacing that suggest that the process has had some undesired side effects. For one thing, many subspecialists appear to be choosing not to take emergency general surgery or trauma call, leading to a potential crisis in our emergency rooms [7]. This is an issue that will definitely require the attention of the profession soon.

Limitations on resident work hours

Beginning July 1, 2003, ACGME mandated that surgical residents were required to work no more than 80 hours per week. Other policies regarding length of work shifts and on-call frequency were instituted simultaneously. The avowed purpose of the new regulations was to improve patient safety by reducing the likelihood of an error committed by a fatigued resident. Because surgical residents in most hospitals had typically worked approximately 100 hours per week before the ACGME mandate, the work hours limitation had the direct effect of limiting residents' direct exposure to patients by about 20%. There have been beneficial effects of the change in terms of resident satisfaction with their personal lives [8], but no plan was in place to replace the educational value of the lost hours or to make the remaining training time more efficient. Residents are generally not used to "homework" assignments, nor does the profession have any significant ability to simulate the clinical environment outside the hospital to allow off-duty residents to hone their clinical skills.

In Europe, legislation adopted by the European Union (EU) currently limits resident works hours in member nations to 58 hours per week. The legislation will require the reduction of work hours to 48 per week by the year 2009. Resident work hours in Canada vary by province, but generally are close to those in the United States. In Canada, however, work hour schedules are negotiated between resident provincial unions and the provincial government. Whether the United States will follow the example of either Canada or the EU is not yet clear. There has not been a rigorous examination of the number of hours required to train the types of surgeons we need in the United States, and this is a study in which the profession might wish to engage. Absent such an examination, work hour limits may be imposed based on superficial arguments, strictly noneducational considerations, or political pressure.

Competency of graduating surgical residents

There is currently a perception in the profession that today's residency graduates are not as capable as those of a generation ago. It is difficult to substantiate this belief, but it seems pervasive. Today's residents have a higher pass rate on ABS examinations than their predecessors, but direct comparison is difficult, because the examinations have changed over time. The certifying (oral) examination, which aims to test clinical skills and judgment, has a more formalized grading process than in the past, and the questions are much more standardized than they were when today's older surgeons took the examination.

Even if the competence of today's graduating residents compared with their predecessors is open to question, there is no doubt that the training is much different. In addition to the reduced hours of direct patient exposure, today's residents are much more heavily supervised and have less (if any) independent operative experience. Independent action, which was the mark of a senior resident a generation ago, is rightfully viewed with skepticism today, but there is a distinct possibility that today's residents are having decisions made for them (by attending surgeons), and may not even realize that a decision was necessary. If so, the resident leaves training unprepared when confronted with the need to make a judgment.

Much of the problem of inexperience could be dealt with by simulating clinical scenarios. Residents could conceivably learn technical skills as well as accumulate experience in decision-making in safe simulated environments. Early studies demonstrate that skills learned in a simulated setting transfer to real patient care, but the tools for clinical simulation remain relatively impractical, expensive, and primitive at this time. Nevertheless, simulation promises to completely transform surgical education in the coming years, and would be a very appropriate area for government research funding as well as private initiatives.

Response of the profession to issues in graduate surgical education

Although surgeons have always considered training to be an important part of their mission, relatively little attention has been paid to education in comparison with clinical care or research. Unfortunately, many view the education process as a natural by-product of patient care. This is clearly not the case, but this prevalent attitude has impeded efforts to define curriculum, enhance faculty teaching skills, create instructional tools, and other initiatives that are second-nature to educators in other disciplines.

In 2002, Dr. Haile Debas [9] called attention to the beleaguered state of graduate surgical education in his presidential address to the American Surgical Association (ASA), following which the ASA convened a "Blue Ribbon Panel" with representation from the ACS, the ABS, the RRC, and the ASA itself. The panel considered a broad range of issues related to surgical education, deliberated over a period of 20 months, and published its conclusions in January 2005 [10]. These recommendations included, among others

Increasing the number of surgical trainees and establishing a permanent task force to monitor surgical manpower needs

Strengthening the teaching skills of academic faculty and stimulating educational research

Dividing surgical training into basic and advanced levels, leading to an earlier opportunity for specialization/differentiation

Developing a standardized, national curriculum in general surgery

During approximately the same time frame, the ABS created a new standing committee on resident education to examine the curriculum in surgery. The ABS was motivated by the sense among its directors that a significant number of candidates presenting for certification had insufficient knowledge and experience in major relevant areas of surgery, such as complex trauma and complex gastrointestinal operations. It was the opinion of the ABS directors that initiatives to improve resident education should be a coordinated effort of all the major organizations with an interest in and responsibility for surgical GME. As a result, the ABS convened a meeting in November 2004 of representatives of the six stakeholder organizations: ABS, ACS, ASA, RRC, Association of Program Directors in Surgery (APDS) and the Association for Surgical Education (ASE). This group met in Philadelphia and agreed to join forces to work on a standardized national curriculum in surgery, and to create a national Web site for resident education. In addition, the group agreed that a surgeon should be chosen who would be based at the ABS office in Philadelphia and be able to devote full-time attention to surgery GME. The ABS agreed to fund much of the cost for this new position, but other attending organizations were asked to contribute toward the position and subsequently agreed to do so. A search process led to the appointment of author Dr. Richard Bell, who began work August 1, 2006. One of Dr. Bell's first projects was to reconvene the multiorganization task force that met in 2004. Before meeting, the members of the group agreed to adopt the name Surgical Council on Resident Education (SCORE).

A critical first step in building a general surgery curriculum is to define the scope of the specialty [11]. SCORE agreed to endorse a defined list of conditions and diseases and a defined list of categories of operative procedures as being within the scope of general surgery. This list of conditions, diseases, and procedures is organized into 40 subject matter modules and can be examined in full at http://www.SurgicalCORE.org. This list of diseases, conditions, and procedures will form the basis of the curriculum for general surgery training, and is intended to encompass the learning needs of surgery residents between their graduation from medical school and entrance into practice. SCORE is focusing its initial curricular efforts on those residents who enter practice after 5 years of general surgical training, and does not at this time foresee a shortening in the length of training. This list of diseases, conditions, and procedures is intended to be a living document, which will be updated on a regular basis as new procedures are developed and new conditions are recognized, or when certain conditions or procedures are no longer relevant to general surgical training. Using the data that recertifying surgeons provide to ABS, it will be possible in the future to test the curriculum against the actual operative experience of graduates. This will insure that residents receive sufficient training in the procedures that they actually perform in practice, and conversely will assure that residents do not waste educational time learning skills that will not be employed in practice.

The Internet offers new learning opportunities for residents and new teaching opportunities for faculty. SCORE has begun the process of developing a national Web site for general surgery education. The Web site will present integrated text, images, audio, and video, and will link to existing content from other sources such as surgical texts and journals. It will feature case-based learning scenarios. It will be possible for local program directors to add enrichment material to the site. The site will incorporate assessment tools such as mock cases, multiple choice quizzes, and other exercises based on the content. The ABS will initially provide administrative support for this project and assume the Webmaster functions. The majority of the content for the site will be provided by members of the APDS, working through the APDS Curriculum Committee.

The RRC now requires a surgical skills laboratory as part of residency training. In addition, the ACS has started a program to accredit skills laboratories. To optimize the use of these laboratories for general surgery training, a curriculum is required. A surgical skills curriculum task force was initiated by the APDS, which is working jointly with the ACS with the objective of improving resident performance through skills practice, and using assessments of skills to determine "OR readiness" of surgical residents.

The ACS Fundamentals of Surgery curriculum is being developed by the ACS's Division of Education, and is focused on basic cognitive and judgment skills in surgery. It is a tool that first-year residents in all surgical specialties can use to gain clinical skills. It is an extension of the ACS's prior work in defining an essential set of skills for first year residents in surgery. The proposed basic surgery curriculum is case-based, and focuses on specific learning objectives and critical thinking. ACS intends to provide access to cases and the curriculum on a Web site.

The list of challenges for the profession in improving the training of the next generation of surgeons is long. In addition to the curricular efforts outlined above, there needs to be an assessment of the public need for surgeons. It is becoming clear that we face a shortage of surgeons, yet we have been loath to increase our training positions. Whether the current focus on subspecialty training matches the public need is not clear. There is evidence that the lack of surgeons with broad training willing to take call for general surgery and trauma emergencies is becoming a pressing problem. The profession also needs to address the structure of training, and be proactive in defining the work hours and length of training on a rational basis. Compensation for residents is an issue that needs attention in view of the increasing number of residents with families, and the substantial debt that today's residents incur in attending college and medical school, which currently averages about $100,000. Finally, the profession needs to seriously deal with the diminishing attractiveness of surgery as a profession, and the high attrition rate from surgical residencies. For example, we should consider being more flexible in our training requirements so as to allow residents the possibility of interrupting residency for child-raising. Serious efforts in these areas will guarantee that surgical training and the profession of surgery will continue to deserve the highly regarded and sought-after status it has traditionally enjoyed.

References

[1] Halsted WS. The training of the surgeon. Bulletin of the Johns Hopkins Hospital 1904;15: 267–75.

[2] Grillo HC, Edward D. Churchill and the "rectangular" surgical residency. Surgery 2004;136: 947–52.

[3] Sanfey HA, Saalwachter-Schulman AR, Nyhof-Young JM, et al. Influences on medical student career choice: gender or generation? Arch Surg 2006;141:1086–94.

[4] Callcut R, Snow M, Lewis B, et al. Do the best students go into general surgery? J Surg Res 2003;115:69–73.

[5] Accreditation Council on Graduate Medical Education. Graduate medical education data resource book academic year 2004–2005. Chicago: Accreditation Council for Graduate Medical Education; 2005. p. 70.

[6] Birkmeyer JD, Stukel TA, Siewers AE, et al. Surgeon volume and operative mortality in the United States. N Engl J Med 2003;349(22):2117–27.

[7] Institute of Medicine. Hospital-based emergency care: at the breaking point. Washington, DC: National Academies Press; 2006. p. 163–200.

[8] Myers JS, Bellini LM, Morris JB, et al. Internal medicine and general surgery residents' attitudes about the ACGME duty hours regulations: a multicenter study. Acad Med 2006; 81:1052–8.

[9] Debas HT. Surgery: a noble profession in a changing world. Ann Surg 2002;236(3):263–9.

[10] Debas HT, Bass BL, Brennan MF, et al. American Surgical Association Blue Ribbon Committee. American surgical association Blue Ribbon Committee Report on surgical education: 2004. Ann Surg 2005;241(1):1–8.

[11] DaRosa DA, Bell RH Jr. Graduate surgical education redesign: reflections on curriculum theory and practice. Surgery 2004;136:966–74.

ELSEVIER
SAUNDERS

SURGICAL
CLINICS OF
NORTH AMERICA

Surg Clin N Am 87 (2007) 825–836

Certification and Maintenance of Certification in Surgery

Robert S. Rhodes, MD*, Thomas W. Biester, MS

*The American Board of Surgery, 1617 John F. Kennedy Boulevard, Suite 860,
Philadelphia, PA 19103-1847, USA*

The impetus for specialty board certification began in the early 1900s, when concerns about the quality of medical practice paralleled concerns about the quality of medical schools that culminated in the Flexner Report. As with the Flexner Report, many of these concerns arose from within the medical community. The first specialty board, the American Board of Ophthalmology, was incorporated in 1917. Other specialty boards formed in the ensuing decades, with a relatively large number of new boards emerging in the 1930s. At first, many of these new boards functioned in relative isolation, but it soon became apparent that there was a lot to gain by sharing experiences. This led to the formation of the Advisory Board for Medical Specialties in 1933, which in turn became the American Board of Medical Specialties (ABMS) in 1970. Table 1 lists the current 24 member boards of the ABMS, with their dates of incorporation.

The formation of the American Board of Surgery (ABS) was a result of the extraordinary leadership of Graham [1,2]. He was able to successfully navigate some stormy political waters and achieve acceptance of an independent ABS among groups that either opposed its formation or wanted the ABS to be under their control. Those interested in the history of activities within the ABS should also read the early history by Rodman [3] and the more recent history by Griffen [4]. These works detail the changes over time in the methods by which the ABS determined surgeons' qualifications for certification. What has not changed is the ABS commitment to apply the best available standards on an equitable basis.

This article outlines the basis and rationale of current certification, as well as recent changes in certification pathways. It also details two very important events in the evolution of certification: the change from lifetime (indefinite)

---

* Corresponding author.
E-mail address: rrhodes@absurgery.org (R.S. Rhodes).

0039-6109/07/$ - see front matter © 2007 Elsevier Inc. All rights reserved.
doi:10.1016/j.suc.2007.06.004
surgical.theclinics.com

Table 1
ABMS member boards and year in which they were approved

Board	Year
American Board of Ophthalmology	1917
American Board of Otolaryngology	1924
American Board of Obstetrics and Gynecology	1930
American Board of Dermatology	1932
American Board of Orthopaedic Surgery	1935
American Board of Pediatrics	1935
American Board of Psychiatry and Neurology	1935
American Board of Radiology	1935
American Board of Urology	1935
American Board of Internal Medicine	1936
American Board of Pathology	1936
American Board of Surgery	1937
American Board of Neurological Surgery	1940
American Board of Anesthesiology	1941
American Board of Plastic Surgery	1941
American Board of Physical Medicine and Rehabilitation	1947
American Board of Colon and Rectal Surgery	1949
American Board of Preventive Medicine	1949
American Board of Family Practice	1969
American Board of Thoracic Surgery	1970
American Board of Nuclear Medicine	1971
American Board of Allergy and Immunology	1971
American Board of Emergency Medicine	1979
American Board of Medical Genetics	1991

certification to time-limited certification; and, more recently, the advent of Maintenance of Certification (MOC).

The requirements for initial certification

Certification in surgery by the ABS requires satisfactory completion of accredited undergraduate medical education and satisfactory completion of a surgery residency accredited by the Accreditation Council for Graduate Medical Education (ACGME) or the Royal College of Physicians and Surgeons of Canada (RCPSC). Applicants for certification must also present evidence of adequate operative experience in the essential content areas of surgery. Upon approval of their application, these individuals are then admissible to, and must successfully complete the examinations for, certification. The first of these is an 8-hour, multiple-choice qualifying examination (QE) that assesses knowledge in all essential content areas of surgery. The QE, like all ABS multiple-choice examinations, is developed through a multitiered review process that assures a consensus as to each question's appropriateness and correct answer. Psychometrically-valid procedures are then use to assess individual item performance, to assess overall examination reliability, and to establish a passing score [5].

Successful completion of this QE is a prerequisite for admission to the certifying examination (CE), an oral examination in which the candidate is asked to manage a broad sample of cases of common surgical problems. Whereas the QE assesses the candidate's knowledge base, the CE assesses judgment and process thinking. Comparative analyses of candidate's performance on these two types of examinations confirm that they measure different attributes.

Although the certification process does not measure competence as such, it positively correlates with other measures of quality [6], as well as a reduced frequency of adverse state medical board licensure actions [7]. It is not surprising then that patients place great value in certification, and rank it closely behind procedural volume and just ahead of the number of liability suits as the three measures that say "a lot" about quality [8].

Despite this high value given certification, there is increasing concern about the quality and safety of medical care, and thus increasing desire for more information about provider competence and outcomes. Current certification (and recertification) processes assess surgeon qualifications (ie, what they can do) at a time when patients increasingly want to know about knowledge plus values, and want information on individuals' actual performance in practice.

One way of appreciating the relationship of certification relative to the assessment of competence is reflected by Miller's pyramid (Fig. 1) [9]. The four steps in the pyramid represent a hierarchy of metrics that assess performance. The bottom step (Knows) represents current specialty board multiple-choice examinations. The next step (Knows How) is exemplified by oral examinations, particularly those that focus on assessing candidates' understanding of critical processes and their judgment. Despite the current value placed on certification, these first two steps are actually low fidelity simulations, because they do not directly assess performance in a clinical setting.

The third step (Shows How) is somewhat greater fidelity, and might be exemplified by performance on a simulator. These first three steps have a common trait in that they still assess, to a greater or lesser extent, a surgeon's qualifications (ie, what he is capable of doing). The fourth and final step (Does) has the greatest fidelity, because it assesses what the surgeon actually does in practice. This step comes closest to addressing the public's desire to know whether a surgeon is competent. An example of the distinction between qualifications (ie, knowing) versus actual doing might be related to appropriate use of prophylactic antibiotics. An extremely high percentage of surgeons correctly answer this on ABS examinations, yet the percentage estimates of appropriate antibiotic use in practice are often substantially lower.

The emergence and rationale of time-limited certification

Concern with the limitations of indefinite certification and the need for time-limited certification achieved national prominence as early as 1940, when the Commission on Graduate Medical Education argued that the exponential growth in medical knowledge made single, lifetime certification

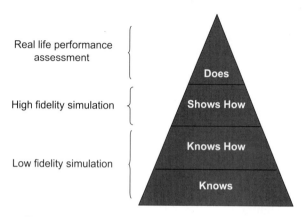

Fig. 1. Miller's pyramid, showing a hierarchy of assessments of competency.

insufficient to assure that individuals kept current in their specialty. Yet time-limited certificates did not become a reality until first adopted by the then American Board of Family Practice (now Family Medicine) in 1970. The ABS instituted 10-year, time-limited certification in pediatric surgery in 1973, the first time-limited surgical certificate (and second overall among ABMS member boards). Since 1976, all ABS certificates have been time-limited.

The ABS now has over 30 years of experience with time-limited certificates, and this considerable experience sheds a great deal of light on the original concerns about maintaining current knowledge. Table 2 shows the fail rates and number of examinees per year for the past 12 years on the recertification examination in surgery, stratified by the number of years since the examinees' initial certification. It is evident that fail rates increase with an increasing number of years since initial certification. Specific failure rates of those first certified in surgery in the years 1991 to 1998, 1981 to 1990, and 1976 to 1980 on the 2006 recertification examination were 4.5%, 6.2%, and 9.4%, respectively.

A particularly notable finding is that fail rates of the 10-year and 20-year cohorts have been relatively constant over time, but fail rates of the 30-year cohort have dropped dramatically since 2003, when diplomates first began to enter this cohort. One possibility to account for the dropping fail rate in this cohort is that the initial 30-year cohorts were simply poor test takers; another is that word of the high fail rates among the initial 30-year examinees has spread and influenced subsequent examinees to better prepare for the examination. A similar trend has been noted in pediatric surgery, which also has 30-year diplomates. Whatever the explanation, these findings corroborate the original concerns about indefinite certification.

This decline in failure rates among the 30-year cohort is encouraging, yet does not tell the whole story, because important differences exist among

Table 2
Number of candidates and the 10-20-30-year ABS diplomate cohort fail rates on the recertification examination in surgery, 1995–2006

	10-year		20-year		30-year		Total	
	#	% F	#	% F	#	% F	#	% F
1995	857	3.6%	252	8.7%	—	—	1109	4.8%
1996	872	4.5%	395	6.8%	—	—	1267	5.2%
1997	830	2.5%	584	7.7%	—	—	1414	4.7%
1998	796	3.0%	678	9.4%	—	—	1474	6.0%
1999	846	3.2%	773	10.5%	—	—	1619	6.7%
2000	639	3.3%	584	12.5%	—	—	1223	7.7%
2001	728	2.6%	642	11.7%	—	—	1370	6.9%
2002	759	4.3%	596	11.9%	—	—	1355	7.7%
2003	816	3.9%	650	16.2%	23	43.5%	1489	9.9%
2004	800	3.8%	665	9.9%	98	22.4%	1563	7.5%
2005	784	4.5%	611	9.3%	160	18.8%	1555	7.8%
2006	753	4.5%	633	6.2%	192	9.4%	1578	5.8%
Total	9480	3.6%	7063	10.3%	473	16.9%	17016	6.8%

Abbreviation: F, fail rate.

some subgroups. One such distinction is that between the interval from initial certification (ie, 10-year, 20-year, 30-year, and so on) and the number of times an individual sought recertification (ie, first, second, or third recertification, and so on). This difference exists because not all surgeons with time-limited certificates have sought to recertify prior to expiration of their certificate. Thus some surgeons may be seeking their first recertification 20-years after their initial certification. Among those are surgeons whose time-limited certificates expired prior to recertification in 2006, for example. The failure rate was 18.0%, versus only 3.3% for those who sought recertification for the first time and were still certificated. This effect is even greater among surgeons whose certificates expired and who missed an entire 10-year recertification cycle. Their overall failure rate was 33%.

Another notable subgroup with significantly higher fail rates are surgeons in solo practice, a finding noted among surgeons certified in surgery and in several subspecialties. The exact reasons for this finding is not clear, but may relate to the relative isolation of these individuals, by choice or design, from relevant peer interactions [10]. A further factor that appears to play a role here was a positive relationship between continuing medical education (CME) activity and examination performance, particularly among surgeons in solo practice [11]. Surgeons in solo practice are also less likely to participate in assessments of practice performance (American Board of Surgery, unpublished data).

In addition to satisfactory performance on a secure examination, specialty board recertification also requires evidence of professionalism (eg, an unrestricted medical license and peer references) and evidence of commitment to lifelong learning (eg, CME activity). The relationship of CME to examination importance was noted above; the significance of assessing professionalism is reflected in findings showing that a high proportion of disciplinary actions by state medical board are related to unprofessional behavior [12]. Unfortunately, the methodological problems of attempting to correlate ABS examination performance with "real-time" performance parameters make it difficult to generate conclusive data on this issue; however, it is known that cognitive errors in judgment or problems with vigilance or memory were contributing factors in 90% of closed malpractice claims [13]. Some surgeons complain that the general nature of the recertification examination is unfair, given that they have a very limited scope of practice. Yet analyses show that many specialists (eg, vascular surgeons, pediatric surgeons, thoracic surgeons) generally do well on the examination despite practicing very little adult general surgery. Moreover, it is not unusual for the individuals who register these complaints to also score poorly on the subtests in their areas of practice focus.

The impetus for broader assessment of physician competence

The limitations of current certification and recertification in assessing competence, together with the Institute of Medicine (IOM) report on medical errors and unnecessary deaths [14], motivated the ABMS member-boards to go beyond the traditional, episodic recertification and explore means of assessing physician competence. Not withstanding the difficulties of defining and measuring competence, the specialty boards, through the ABMS and together with the ACGME, identified six competencies that characterize a competent physician [15]. These competencies and their scopes are listed in Table 3. Most of them are self-evident, and to a certain extent were already assessed as part of traditional episodic recertification. An exception may be systems-based practice, which emphasizes the increasing recognition of the role of the health care team and systems of care, rather than the physician alone, in determining outcomes. These six competencies became the foundation of Maintenance of Certification, a program that consists of four distinct and measurable parts or components (Table 4). Participation in MOC began in 2005, and will be required of all new ABS diplomates and all current ABS diplomates when their current certificates expire.

The specific requirements of each component of MOC will vary among ABMS specialty boards, based on the nature of the specialty and the available tools to assess each component. For the ABS, Parts I through III of MOC will mirror those of traditional recertification, although under MOC, compliance will need to be documented every 3 rather than every 10 years. Part I of MOC, Evidence of Professional Standing, will require maintaining a valid, unrestricted license and peer references. Part II of MOC, Lifelong Learning and Self-assessment, will require the same number

Table 3
The six ABMS/ACGME competencies and their scope

Competency	Scope
Medical knowledge	Evolving biomedical, clinical, and cognate sciences, and the application of this knowledge to patient care
Patient care	Compassionate, appropriate, and effective treatment of health problems and promotion of health
Interpersonal and communication skills	Effective information exchange and teaming with patients, their families, and other health professionals
Professionalism	A commitment to professional responsibilities, adherence to ethical principles, and sensitivity to a diverse patient population
Practice-based learning and improvement	Evaluation of one's own patient care and outcomes, assimilation of scientific evidence, and targeted improvement efforts
Systems-based practice	An awareness of and responsiveness to the systems and environments that affect the delivery of health care, and the ability to best coordinate those systems to provide optimal care

of yearly hours of CME as required for traditional recertification, but they will be required every year rather than the 2 years prior to the examination. The specific requirement is 50 hours of CME per year, 30 of which must be Category I. This level of CME activity corresponds to the 100 hours of CME, including 60 Category I credits, heretofore required during the 2 years preceding the application for traditional recertification.

A further change in Part II will be an increasing emphasis on self-assessment rather than conventional CME. Such self-assessment requires surgeons to be more actively engaged in the learning process, and to provide feedback on what they have learned. The rationale for this emphasis is evidence that traditional CME requires learner feedback or peer reinforcement to produce practice change [16–18].

MOC will also increasingly emphasize self-assessment of cognitive expertise. In general, approved self-assessment activities will meet the requirement for CME, but all CME activities may not involve self-assessment. The American College of Surgeons (ACS) Self Education and Self-Assessment Program (SESAP) is an example of an acceptable self-assessment activity. Because the availability of suitable self-assessment activities may be limited, the ABS is encouraging development of additional resources by surgical specialty societies. An encouraging development in this regard is the approval of new formats for CME credit, to include performance improvement, internet searching and learning, and journal-based activities [19]. Acceptable

Table 4
The four parts of ABS MOC and their respective activities

Part	MOC component	ABS requirement
I	Evidence of Professional Standing	• Possession of a valid, full, and unrestricted medical license • Reference letters to be submitted from the chief of surgery and chair of credentialing/privileges committee of the institution where the majority of work is performed
II	Commitment to Lifelong Learning and Self-assessment	• 30 hours of Category I and 20 hours of Category II CME to be performed yearly • Self-assessment evaluation in conjunction with CME to be performed and verified every third year, through the American College of Surgeons' Surgical Education and Self-Assessment Program (SESAP) or other acceptable self-assessment tools as developed
III	Evidence of Cognitive Expertise	• Successful completion of a secure examination at 10-year intervals, offered beginning in the seventh year after certification or recertification
IV	Evaluation of Performance in Practice	• Participation in a national, regional, or local surgical outcomes study or quality assessment program, including patient communication skills assessment, with verification every third year of MOC. Peer review may also be used if adequate assessment programs are not available.

self-assessment activities are posted on the ABS Web site, www.absurgery. org/default.jsp?exam-moc., and will be periodically updated.

Part III of MOC, Evidence of Cognitive Expertise, will be the same as the current secure examination, although an implication of multiple cycles of the other components of MOC within the 10-year recertification cycle is that the successful completion of the examination in the 7- to 10-year window will not necessarily be the final step in recertification.

The biggest change in MOC over traditional recertification is the addition of Part IV, Assessment of Practice Performance. This is a shift from measuring an individual's qualifications toward measuring competence. The philosophical cornerstone of Part IV is that improvement requires measurement. Although there is some concern with the validity of such measurements for making provider comparisons, a key point is that the intent is to use performance data for improvement rather than judgment. Moreover, the emphasis will be on evidence-based process measures (eg, timing of preoperative antibiotics) or outcomes (eg, wound infections).

This emphasis on process measures will overcome many of the problems associated with outcome assessments. These problems include the often unpredictable nature of patients' responses to treatment, the statistical issues of analyzing a relatively small number of patients with a given procedure within a surgeon's practice, and the inability to adequately adjust for differences in severity. A key aspect of assessment of performance is that it will be a multistage process; subsequent steps will include the development and implementation of an improvement model, which is then to be followed by reassessment of performance.

Recognized methodological shortcomings of assessing individual surgeon outcomes include difficulties in identifying statistical differences among relatively small numbers and in adjusting for differences in the severity of illness. Moreover, for a number of complex surgical procedures, hospital volume may play as significant a role as surgeon volume and experience. Systems of care within the institution are likely to be important in these circumstances. Thus, the ABS will also accept valid measures of institutional outcomes. Perhaps the best known of such measures is the National Surgical Quality Improvement Program (NSQIP). This was initially an endeavor within the Veterans Administration (VA) hospital system, but has now been extended to non-VA facilities by the ACS [20]. Although NSQIP assesses institutional rather than individual surgeon outcomes, the likelihood is that some of the factors affecting such outcomes are a result of institutional systems. As with the self-assessment activities in Part II, a list of acceptable practice performance assessment activities will be regularly updated on the ABS Web site.

Although having to complete three cycles of assessment of practice performance (one cycle every 3 years) during the 10-year MOC cycle may seem onerous, recent surveys of diplomates seeking recertification show that about one half of them already participate in some form of outcomes assessment (American Board of Surgery, unpublished data, 2006). The ABS will also make every attempt to align its requirements for assessment of practice performance with those of other organizations (eg, participation in a state or Medicare pay-for-performance/physician quality reporting initiative [21]).

Special circumstances

Two special circumstances may affect one's participation in MOC. The first will involve the approximately 20% of surgeons who initially certify in surgery and then subsequently certify in another ABS or ABMS specialty. To facilitate MOC participation among individuals with multiple certificates, the ABS will credit evidence of Professional Standing, Lifelong Learning and Self-assessment, and Assessment of Practice Performance (Parts I, II, and IV of MOC) that complies with any other ABS or ABMS-member board MOC program as compliant with the ABS MOC program.

The assessment of Cognitive Expertise by a secure examination (Part III) will still be necessary in all disciplines in which the diplomate is certified.

The second circumstance involves surgeons who are clinically inactive but wish to remain certified. This is a complex issue, because Assessment of Practice Performance (Part IV of MOC) may not be relevant to such individuals. In such cases, the ABS will waive the requirement for Part IV, but to avoid misleading the public as to the equivalence of such certification, will mark these certificates as "clinically inactive," and will so report this status to all who inquire.

The benefits and future of maintenance of certification

As noted above, MOC was created in response to increasing concerns about the quality and safety of medical care, and the increasing desire for accountability among the medical profession. These concerns were reinforced by a subsequent study that found that appropriate care was provided only slightly more than half the time [22], and another study that presented evidence of a relationship between decreases in practice performance and the duration of practice [23].

The ABS firmly believes that both patients and physicians stand to benefit from MOC. Patients will benefit from improvements in quality and safety, and physicians will benefit from the increased awareness of the quality of their practice. Presently only about one in three physicians appear to receive any data (process, outcome, or patient surveys) about the quality of care they provide [24]. Given that the Evaluation of Performance in Practice (Part IV of MOC) assessments of practice performance will be external measures (eg, participation in NSQIP, participation in the Surgical Care Improvement Project [SCIP]), the benefits of MOC will not come from MOC as such, but from the increased level of surgeon participation in these activities. With time, it will become evident that some performance assessment activities are more effective in improving the quality of care than others; the acceptability of specific activities toward fulfilling the requirements for MOC will change accordingly.

An additional benefit to surgeons will be the enhanced public trust that results from their willingness to assess their practice. Physician concerns about quality of care were the original impetus for specialty board certification. Rededication to improving quality of care through a physician-led specialty board will allow surgeons to address public concerns about the quality and safety of health care and simultaneously recapture public perceptions of physician expertise and authority.

Undoubtedly, some diplomates may consider MOC to be both burdensome and intrusive. Yet even without MOC, such activities are increasingly likely to be required by health care purchasers or governmental agencies. MOC will enhance the meaning of board certification as a standard of quality and physicians' commitment to continual practice improvement and lifelong learning. Given this situation, physicians should not underestimate the greater value attached to assessments that come from physician-led organizations.

There are also concerns that the amount of time and effort related to measuring the myriad of potentially measurable processes in health care could easily overwhelm time for actual patient care. Sustained improvement will require a much greater reliance on information technology and related infrastructure, and this is likely to take many years to evolve. Yet despite such barriers, physicians must be engaged in this effort now even while MOC is a work in progress. Physicians are the only stakeholders in this effort with sufficient expertise to address quality issues; voluntarily doing so is likely to go a long way toward reducing pressure for mandated, burdensome, or intrusive actions.

Although it is important to remember that MOC focuses on specific competencies, it is possible that assessing surgeon competence may continue to be difficult to define and measure. This is because surgical judgments are complex and will always include some degree of uncertainty. Moreover, ongoing rapid advances in knowledge and technology also make quality a moving target. Indeed, nearly 100 years ago Ernest Codman said: "The science of medicine, however, sophisticated it may be, is always in the experimental stage" [25]. Codman's observation that we are all in the business of quality improvement is even more relevant today than in his time.

Summary

ABS certification traditionally assessed surgeons' qualifications, but the concerns about quality and safety are placing increasing demands to assess how surgeons actually perform in practice. The ABS MOC program is designed to require periodic assessments of practice performance in addition to the current measures used for certification and recertification. The degree to which surgeons accept and meet this challenge is likely to have important implications for both public perceptions of the profession and future health policy.

References

[1] Mueller CB. Evarts A. Graham: the life, lives, and times of the surgical spirit of St. Louis. Hamilton (BC): Decker, Inc; 2002. p. 220–29.

[2] Ravitch M. A century of surgery: 1880–1980, vol. II, appendix C, Philadelphia: JB Lippincott Co.; 1981. p.1542–6.

[3] Rodman JS. History of the American Board of Surgery: 1937–1952. Philadelphia: JB Lipincott Co.; 1956.

[4] Griffen WO. The American Board of Surgery in the 20th century: then and now. Philadelphia: American Board of Surgery; 2004.

[5] Rhodes RS, Biester TW, Bell RH, et al. Assessing surgical knowledge: a primer on the examination policies of the American Board of Surgery. J Surg Educ 2007;64:138–42.

[6] Brennan TA, Horwitz RI, Duffy FD, et al. The role of physician specialty board certification status in the quality movement. JAMA 2004;292:1038–43.

[7] Kohatsu ND, Gould D, Ross LK, et al. Characteristics associated with physician discipline; a case controlled study. Arch Intern Med 2004;164:653–8.

[8] The Henry J. Kaiser Family Foundation. National survey on consumers' experiences with patient safety and quality information—survey and chartpack. 2004. Available at: http://www.kff.org/kaiserpolls/7209.cfm. Accessed January 27, 2007.

[9] Miller GE. The assessment of clinical skills/competence/performance. Acad Med 1990; 65(9 Suppl):S63–7.

[10] St. George IM. Professional isolation and performance: a case-control study. Journal of Medical Licensure and Discipline 2006;92:12–5.

[11] Rhodes RS, Biester TW, Malangoni M, et al. Continuing medical education activity and American Board of Surgery examination performance. J Am Coll Surg 2003;196:604–10.

[12] Khaliq AA, Dimassi H, Hiang CY, et al. Disciplinary action against physicians: who is likely to get disciplined? Am J Med 2005;118:773–7.

[13] Rogers SO, Gawande AA, Kwaan M, et al. Analysis of surgical errors in closed malpractice claims at 4 liability insurers. Surgery 2006;140:25–33.

[14] Institute of Medicine. To err is human: building a safer health system. Washington, DC: National Academy Press; 1999.

[15] Steinbrook R. Renewing board certification. N Engl J Med 2005;353(19):1994–7.

[16] Davis DA, Thomson MA, Oxman AD, et al. Changing physician performance: a systematic review of the effect of continuing medical education strategies. JAMA 1995;274:700–5.

[17] Davis DA, O'Brien MJT, Freemantle N, et al. Impact of formal continuing medical education: do conferences, workshops, rounds or other traditional activities change physician behavior or outcomes? JAMA 1999;282:867–74.

[18] Mazmanian PE, Davis DA. Continuing medical education and the physician as learner: guide to the evidence. JAMA 2002;288:1057–60.

[19] The Accreditation Council for Continuing Medical Education. Available at: http://www.accme.org/dir_docs/doc_upload/fd31627e-1510-4e6f-90bb-67b0adca2c38_uploaddocument.pdf. Accessed March 27, 2006.

[20] The American College of Surgeons. Available at: http://www.facs.org/cqi/outcomes.html. Accessed March 20, 2006.

[21] Centers for Medicare and Medicaid Services. Available at: http://www.cms.hhs.gov/PQRI/. Accessed January 22, 2007.

[22] McGlynn EA, Asch SM, Adams J, et al. The quality of health care in the United States. N Engl J Med 2003;348:2635–45.

[23] Choudry NK, Fletcher RH, Soumerai SB. Systematic review: the relationship between clinical experience and the quality of health care. Ann Intern Med 2005;142:260–73.

[24] Audet A-MJ, Doty MM, Shamasdin J, et al. Measure, learn, improve; physician's involvement in quality improvement. Health Aff 2005;24:843–53.

[25] Codman EA. Re-engineering clinical records for production control: 1917. Aust Health Rev 2001;24:71–3.

ELSEVIER
SAUNDERS

SURGICAL
CLINICS OF
NORTH AMERICA

Surg Clin N Am 87 (2007) 837–852

Assessing the Quality of Surgical Care

Aaron S. Fink, MD[a],*, Kamal M. Itani, MD[b],
Darrell C. Campbell, Jr, MD[c]

[a]Department of Surgery, Emory University School of Medicine and Surgical Service,
VAMC—Atlanta, 1670 Clairmont Road (112), Decatur, GA 30033, USA
[b]Boston Veterans Administration Healthcare System and Boston University, Boston Medical
Center and Brigham and Women's Hospitals, Boston, MA, USA
[c]The University of Michigan Hospitals and Health Centers, Ann Arbor, MI, USA

Following the Institute of Medicine's description of the "quality chasm" [1,2], safety and quality have become prominent criteria by which surgical care is evaluated. Surgeons and hospitals are increasingly asked for evidence addressing these areas. Such demands arise from a better educated clientele and more demanding payers, as well as regulatory agencies. Patients and families are using this documentation to select their surgical practitioners and the sites for their care. In addition, payers are seeking to use the data to direct selected patient populations to particular providers, and potentially to adjust reimbursement rates [3]. Therefore, health care policy makers, health service researchers, and others are aggressively seeking to develop and implement quality indicators that can be appropriately applied to surgical practice.

According to Donabedian [4,5], inferences about the quality of care can be drawn from three components: structure, process, and outcome. Structure refers to the material, human, and organization attributes of the particular health care setting. Process refers to both the patient's activities in seeking care and the practitioner's activities in providing same. Finally, outcome denotes the effects of the rendered care on the health status of the patient or the population. Donabedian [4] noted that although these components are integrally related, such relationships must be established before any particular element can be used to assess quality of care. As he so eloquently stated, "There must be pre-existing knowledge of the linkage between structure and process, and between process and outcome, before quality assessment can be undertaken" [4].

* Corresponding author.
E-mail address: aaron.fink@va.gov (A.S. Fink).

0039-6109/07/$ - see front matter © 2007 Elsevier Inc. All rights reserved.
doi:10.1016/j.suc.2007.06.002
surgical.theclinics.com

Factors germane to each of the components have been used as quality and safety metrics. Although elements within each category have been adopted by different bodies and agencies, each has associated advantages and disadvantages [6]. Structural features and process measures within an institution are easy to measure, and yet often seem unrelated to outcomes. That is to say, they lack face validity. Outcomes measurements, in contrast, have great face validity, but are difficult and time-consuming to collect.

As surgeons, we harbor a responsibility to participate in the development and deployment of any measures by which our care will be evaluated [7]. Thus, in this brief overview, the authors address the three components described by Donabedian and discuss their potential merit as quality indicators. Ultimately, surgeons must work collaboratively with payers, health organizations, and regulatory agencies to develop hybrid systems that best support our common goals—decreasing morbidity and mortality while improving the overall quality of surgical care.

Structure

Systems and structures play a critical role in the final outcome of surgical care. Structural measures include a very broad group of variables that reflect the setting in which care is delivered; their delineation ultimately describes the system and resources that are available to support the health care provided.

Within the context of outcomes, one invariably encounters multiple subsystems that address single tasks. Compilation of these subsystems, in turn, can be viewed as simple systems, many of which interact to create complex systems. The larger systems interact with each other to create a more complex system: an organization. The organization is a structure that holds the interacting subsystems, systems, and complex systems together. The organization's structure can be rigid or dynamic, depending on the culture, the need for change and improvement, and the availability of resources.

Medical systems are distinctive with respect to complexity of content and organizational structure. Whereas nonmedical systems are typically managed vertically through hierarchical control, patient care systems tend to comprise numerous diverse components that are loosely aggregated [8]. Within patient care systems, subsystems (including quality improvement components) tend to function in isolation, and structural changes tend to be managed laterally across individual systems. All too often, the latter situation results in ineffective or even contradictory policies, thereby increasing the chances of poor outcome [9]. Because patient care routine involves multiple individuals within simple, bigger, or complex systems, changing routines to reliably improve patient outcome will require that structural changes occur across and between those groups and divisions [10].

Unlike process measures, which can often be evaluated in randomized clinical trials, most structural measures can only be assessed in observational studies. In addition, structural variables reflect average results for large groups of institutions rather than individual surgeons. Therefore, as noted by Donabedian [4,5], the observation of outcomes is an indirect means of assessing the overall structure of care.

Some of the best tools available for measuring outcome at the federal, state, regional, and local levels make use of proprietary and publicly available risk-adjustments systems. Although the National Surgical Quality Improvement Project (NSQIP) is discussed in greater detail later in this article, it is pertinent to note that as a means of validating this risk-adjusted outcome assessment system, site visits of the 10 hospitals with the highest and lowest risk-adjusted morbidity and mortality were conducted. During these site visits, significant differences in various structural parameters (Box 1) were noted between the two groups [11]. By way of example, the site visit teams rated low-outliers significantly higher than high-outliers for the "technology and equipment dimension." Team ratings on the other six dimensions were consistently higher for low-outlier hospitals, although these differences reached only borderline statistical significance [11]. These findings support the NSQIP's role as a tool by which possible structural concerns within a hospital or health care system can be identified.

Associations between risk-adjusted mortality rates and structures of surgical care have also been explored outside the Veterans Administration (VA) system in cardiac surgery [12,13] and intensive care units [14]. In all of these reports, there was a significant association between improvement of structural variables and subsequent improved performance. Other examples of successful structural changes leading to improved outcomes have been documented by both the Intermountain Health System in Utah [15] and the Maine Medical Assessment Foundation [16]. These structural changes shared four important characteristics: (1) providers responded to practice variations by participating in outcomes research; (2) voluntary physician-initiated interventions were as effective as, if not more effective than, external regulatory mechanisms in reducing mortality and morbidity;

Box 1. Structural parameters assessed by the National Surgical Quality Improvement Project in high- and low-outlier hospitals

Technology and equipment
Technical competence
Interface with other services
Relationship with affiliated institutions
Monitoring of quality of care
Coordination of work
Leadership
Overall quality of care

(3) a systems approach to quality improvement produce better results than a bad-apple approach; and (4) quality improvement programs successfully included groups that otherwise might have been competitors [9].

Another potential structural variable that has received significant attention is the relationship between surgical volume and outcome [17,18]. It is presumed that, partly as a result of the higher procedural volumes in certain hospitals, structural systems have developed to safely accommodate such case volumes and obtain improved outcomes. Unfortunately, many of these data are based on observational studies using administrative databases poorly adjusted for case mix [19]. In addition, serious methodological limitations of the relationship between volume and outcome have been raised [20–22]. Indeed, the same argument can be made about structural systems supporting complex surgeries within small-volume hospitals; although those structures are not routinely present in low-volume hospitals, the heightened alertness and vigilance implemented when performing complex surgeries may prevent errors and result in a good outcome. This premise is supported by the fact that presumptive volume-outcome relationships based on administrative databases have not been substantiated by prospectively collected and risk-adjusted data such as the NSQIP [23,24]. Although there is little doubt that volume at the individual surgeon level is important [25], higher-volume surgeons can perform poorly in systems with poor structures, and lower-volume surgeons can perform well in systems with strong structures [6,9,11]. Exceptions may include complex surgeries such as pancreaticoduodenectomies, esophagectomies, and coronary artery bypass [26,27], in which surgeon experience and structural support at the institutional level do seem to be important for good outcome, supporting a potential volume-outcome relationship for these procedures [18].

Undoubtedly, the best way to assess and understand structural variables is to site-visit the system in question. Such visits might be appropriate for a hospital or health care system identified as a high-outlier for overall or specialty-specific risk-adjusted mortality or morbidity, or with a specific problem such as high rates of surgical site infection or postoperative myocardial infarction. These visits should be designed to assess variables such as those listed in Box 1, or other structural parameters relevant to the issue in question.

Although such visits are usually expensive and time-consuming, they allow for the assessment and identification of system issues in high-outliers. The site visits would also help in the elimination of confounding issues as an explanation for observed associations between structure and outcomes. As alluded to above, since its inception, the VA NSQIP has used a well-defined site visit strategy (Table 1) and visited high-outliers for risk-adjusted mortality. Low-outlier facilities have also been visited, so that information about identified model systems can be disseminated through the outcome-based annual reports. High-outlier facilities can learn from low-outlier facilities as well as from comments and suggestions made during the site visit.

Table 1
Level of concern triggering a paper audit or site review in the NSQIP

Level 0.5	There is a high O/E mortality ratio for at least one subspecialty but not all operations in the current fiscal year	Recommend paper audit of all surgical deaths
Level 1.0	There is a high O/E mortality ratio for all operations and/or all noncardiac operations in the current fiscal year	Recommend paper audit of all surgical deaths
Level 2.0	There is a high O/E mortality ratio for all operations and/or all noncardiac operations in the current fiscal year and one additional period in the past 4 years	Recommend follow-up report and/ or site visit
Level 3.0	There is a high O/E mortality ratio for all operations and/or all noncardiac operations in the current fiscal year and two or more other periods in the past 4 years	Recommend follow-up report and/ or site visit

Processes of care

In the paradigm of quality articulated by Donabedian [4,5], processes of care fall between structural measurements and outcomes measurements. Process measurements, which reflect the care patients actually receive, have some face validity and are easier to measure than outcomes. For these reasons, processes of care have recently received greater attention than either structural elements or outcomes measurements.

The interest in processes of care has increased because they allow more targeted actions than either structural elements or outcomes measurements. By way of example, although an unacceptably high surgical mortality might demand more attention, such an undesired outcome may well be attributable to a wide variety of problems in surgical care delivery, none of which are immediately obvious. Although actionable, focusing on a specific process in the perioperative period requires confidence that the chosen process is tightly linked to the high mortality rate. Unfortunately, the evidence linking various surgical processes of care to outcomes is quite limited at present and demands much further study. Clearly, such studies require a validated and standardized outcome metric, as is described later.

The processes of care of most interest to health care systems are those that can be applied to large patient populations. When applied rigorously, such processes could have a large impact on overall results. Examples include optimal deep venous thrombosis (DVT) prophylaxis, tight postoperative glycemic control, and proper administration of perioperative antibiotics. What has not been as well-studied are areas involving specific surgical procedures. For various reasons, including the lack of a standard-ized outcome metric, even the most basic processes are not supported by evidence. For example, despite the over 60-year history of colon surgery, we remain uncertain whether preoperative bowel cleansing—the standard bowel preparation—is advantageous or not [28].

The medical community is rushing to provide actionable process measures that can be targeted for quality improvement and are reportable to various external agencies and the public. Further, the enthusiasm of the federal gov-ernment, payers, and the public for pay-for-performance—much of which will be based on process measure compliance—has outpaced any evidence linking selected process measures, even those with at least some evidence base, to the desired outcomes. Although this interest is understandable, many of the process measures selected for scrutiny have not yet been properly validated and field tested (eg, normothermia in colorectal surgery). This fact presents a considerable problem: the public wants to know but the doctors have little faith in the metric.

As an example of how process measures can be launched into prominence prematurely, when linkage of acute myocardial infarction to cardiovascular outcomes were actually studied nationally, adherence to the CORE mea-sures only accounted for 6% of the variance in cardiovascular outcomes [29]. These data suggest that there are a wide variety of other critical pro-cesses yet to be discovered in this area.

Another example from the surgical community involves the Agency for Health Care Research and Quality (AHRQ) Patient Safety Indicators (PSI). The PSI consists of 20 indicators generated from administrative data sources (billing data) for assessing processes of care. One of the indicators, retained foreign objects following surgery, would seem to be the most basic indicator imaginable for surgery. Yet when initial validation studies were done (after the release of the PSI), it was discovered that the indicator actu-ally captured surgical drains intentionally left in place or surgical sponges initially missed on the first sponge count but successfully retrieved before the second count and extubation. No surgeon would consider the latter case to represent a retained sponge, but computers are not surgeons, and if reported without correction, the metric would reflect unfairly on the institu-tions' processes of care. Indeed, in this example, the process of care correctly identified the problem and functioned superbly. These are the types of "glitches" in the reporting system that need to be identified; that is, the metric needs to be validated before implementation. Following such validation studies, the metrics should be field tested in a variety of pilot sites to further establish reliability, credibility, and optimal logistics of implementation.

Processes of care measurement

Measurement systems for surgical processes of care reached the forefront of attention with the Surgical Infection Prevention Project (SIP), a joint effort of the Centers for Disease Control and Prevention (CDC) and of Centers for Medicare and Medicaid Services (CMS). SIP established three performance measures in the area of surgical infection. SIP 1 focused on timing of antibiotic administration before incision (within 60 minutes); SIP 2 focused on the use of the correct antibiotic choice based on circumstance; whereas SIP 3 was aimed not at infection prevention, but at the increasing emergence of antibiotic-resistant organisms in surgery (discontinuation of antibiotics within 24 hours postoperatively) [30,31]. The effectiveness of this approach was recognized by the National Surgical Infection Prevention Collaborative. As shown in Table 2, the 12-month effort, involving 34,133 patients, resulted in substantial improvement in all three areas of interest. More importantly, the overall incidence of operative site infection decreased by 27% [32].

Following the SIP initiative and endorsement of these measures by the Joint Commission on Accreditation of Healthcare Organizations (JCAHO), CMS expanded its effort by developing the Surgical Care Improvement Project (SCIP) which bundled the three SIP measures with several additional measures addressing surgical site infection (glucose control for cardiac surgical patients, appropriate hair removal at the surgical site, and immediate postoperative normothermia for colorectal surgical patients). In addition to infection prevention, other process measures added to SCIP included the use of perioperative beta blockers to prevent adverse myocardial outcomes, and prophylaxis for deep venous thrombosis. SCIP's overall goal is a 25% reduction in the incidence of surgical complications by the year 2010 [33].

Although SCIP is a noble effort, implementation problems have arisen because of the previously mentioned lack of a robust evidence base. As an example, the use of perioperative beta-blockers was questioned for general surgical patients when a large meta-analysis documented an inadequate number of patients in randomized clinical trials to firmly demonstrate a benefit for an intervention that imposed substantial risk of bradycardia and hypotension [34]. This analysis caused the American College of Cardiology to withdraw its support for this SCIP measure in the context of general surgical patients.

Table 2
Progressive improvement by quarter of the National Surgical Infection Prevention Collaborative compared with baseline established by national sample

Performance measure	National baseline (%)	Median performance by quarter (%)			
		1st	2nd	3rd	4th
Antibiotic ≤60 min	56	72	82	89	92
Correct antibiotic	92.6	90	94	95	95
Discontinued ≤24 h	40.7	67	79	74	85

Data from Fry DE. The surgical infection prevention project: processes, outcomes, and future impact. Surg Infect (Larchmt) 2006;7:S24.

Problems notwithstanding, the federal government has enthusiastically supported SIP and SCIP. Hospitals not reporting SIP measure compliance currently face a 0.4% reduction in Medicare payments. In addition, the Deficit Reduction Act of 2005 requires compliance with 17 process and outcomes measures [35]. Failure to report on these measures will result in a 2% penalty in Medicare payment [36]. Currently, these stipulations only involve penalties for nonreporting, but no one doubts that pay-for-performance, based at least in part on SCIP measures, is around the corner. Indeed, although not yet policy, many have suggested that over the next several years, CMS will withhold payments for hospital-acquired infections.

No studies linking SCIP measures with risk-adjusted surgical site infection (SSI) outcomes have been reported or are likely to occur before real money is awarded for SCIP measure compliance. As further discussed below, the existing studies are flawed by their use of administrative data sets, which only record events occurring during the index hospitalization [37]. Unfortunately, most wound infections occur long after the patient has been discharged; as such, many such events are not recorded as complications, limiting the usefulness of this approach. It will be difficult to establish a tight linkage of any SCIP measure to outcomes in the absence of more reliable data. This shortfall will generate frustration among physicians and other providers, and may prevent future development of more important indicators.

As discussed in the next section, more reliable surgical outcomes data do exist in the form of the VA and the American College of Surgeons' (ACS)-NSQIP. In contrast to administrative data sets, the NSQIP methodology allows capture of most wound infections occurring within the first 30 days postoperatively, and thus provides a more accurate reflection of any preventive process of care. Any SCIP measure's strength would be greatly enhanced were it to be linked to a specific ACS-NSQIP clinical outcome. If such a linkage were demonstrated (ie, adherence to the measure is associated with a favorable risk-adjusted outcome), a measure should be continued. If no important linkage can be shown, it should be discontinued and others should be developed and then tested. A preliminary effort to link structural elements and processes of care with outcomes has come out of the recently completed Patient Safety in Surgery study [38,39], described in the next section.

Outcomes

Surgical procedures involve an intervention with an expected outcome—an inguinal hernia repair is expected to proceed without mortality or complication (eg, infection), and to result in a stable repair that does not deteriorate over time. Thus, given the nature of surgical interventions, outcomes are particularly appealing as measures of surgical quality. Ideally, outcomes used in evaluating a particular intervention would be either the frequency of complete and permanent cure of the illness being treated, or a comparison of the patient's functional status before or after intervention.

Although this information may be ascertained under certain circumstances, such data are not currently available in the general health setting for all patients. As a result, broader outcome measures have been used, including mortality, morbidity (either global or specific), readmission rates, and so on.

Comparisons of such outcome metrics among individuals or institutions are typically held to portray quality of surgical care. Such comparisons are often compromised, however, by the divergent risk profiles associated with the patient population in question [40,41]. Failure to recognize such patient-related factors ignores their potential impact on treatment response. Further, comparisons made without completely adjusting for such divergent risk profiles may hide serious quality issues at institutions treating low-risk patients, while causing providers of care to high-risk patients to appear inferior [41]. Indeed, without adequate risk-adjustment schema, attempts to improve surgical quality based on unadjusted data could actually result in the opposite effect. Fearing selective contracting or reimbursement adjustments, outlier physicians might refuse to treat high-risk patients or "upcode" morbid conditions. Such concerns emphasize the import of adequate and validated risk-adjustment measures, developed with and supported by provider involvement.

As noted by Iezzoni [41], most of the earliest risk-adjustment systems sought to trade off detailed, clinical risk assessments for logistical feasibility and reasonable cost. As a result, most of these early systems (eg, Computerized Severity Index [CSI], MedisGroups, DiseaseStaging) were based on limited clinical information of questionable accuracy, a problem that continues to influence most of the systems depending solely upon administrative data [37,41–43].

As hospital costs began to increase in the 1980s, demand increased for more accurate methods by which to risk-adjust for illness severity, and thereby more accurately confirm the value of local hospital care [41]. The "buy right" experiment, lead by Walter McClure in Minneapolis, typified such early efforts [41]. McClure [44], who believed that clinically credible data were essential to valid risk-adjustment, noted that, "There is no other way than to go in and abstract the clinical findings from the chart. Let's stop fooling ourselves that we can compare patient severity by claims."

Several new initiatives that used clinical information from medical records to risk-adjust hospital mortality rates (eg, Cleveland Health Quality Choice [45], Department of Veterans Affairs Surgical Risk Study [NVASRS] [11,46–48], Northern New England Cardiovascular Disease Study Group [13]) appeared soon thereafter. As the clinical databases within these systems grew, empirical techniques were used to refine severity measures. In addition, the systems were able to develop different models for predicting different outcomes. Such capabilities and refinements afforded scientific rigor and clinical credibility to this new generation of severity measures. Unfortunately, these systems, which are so dependent on medical record abstraction, proved costly [49]. As a result, because of the projected costs of application,

many of these initiatives were halted and discharge abstract-based measures
were adopted or readopted instead [41].

Ongoing concerns about the accuracy and credibility of administratively
based measures persisted [50,51]. In 1993, the Health Care Financing
Administration (HCFA, now CMS), which had published hospital mortality
rates since 1986, discontinued such publication, citing the inaccuracy of
their abstract-based risk-adjustment methodology—especially for inner-
city public hospitals [52]. Concerns about data quality forced California
to conduct a special study about data accuracy [53]. Regulatory agencies
were left to decide between two options: providing funds to abstract clinical
data from medical records, or relying upon review of administrative data
[41].

The National Surgical Quality Improvement Project

Conducted between 1991 and 1993 in response to a 1985 Congressional
mandate [54], the National VA Surgical Risk Study (NVASRS) aimed to
develop and validate risk-adjustment models for the prediction of surgical
outcome, and the comparative assessment of the quality of surgical care
among different facilities [11,46–48]. As noted above, medical record abstraction was used in developing risk-adjustment models for 30-day mortality and morbidity rates for all noncardiac surgery, and for each of multiple
surgical subspecialties (general surgery, vascular surgery, orthopedic surgery, urology, neurosurgery, noncardiac thoracic surgery, plastic surgery,
and otolaryngology). After demonstrating the applicability of the NVASRS
models and validating their ability to detect variations in the quality of surgical care, the Department of Veterans Affairs (DVA) provided funding to
establish the NSQIP, applying the methodology developed in the NVASRS
to all 132 Veterans Affairs Medical Centers performing surgery across the
nation [49]. In doing so, the DVA established a reporting and managerial
structure by which surgical quality could be monitored and improved within
the Veterans Health Administration (VHA) [49,55,56].

The NSQIP methodology has been extensively reviewed in previous publications [46–49,55]. Briefly, at each VA hospital performing major surgery,
both workload (case volume categorized by specialty and "major or minor"
classification, including Current Procedural Terminology [CPT] codes) and
risk-adjustment (45 preoperative, 17 intraoperative, and 33 outcome variables) data are collected by a dedicated, trained surgical clinical nurse reviewer. Uniformity is maintained by use of an operations manual detailing
data-collection processes and variable definitions, as well as regularly scheduled conference calls with all nurse reviewers.

The risk-adjustment data are entered by the nurse reviewer into a special
risk-adjustment software module, integrated into the surgical module of the
VA's decentralized hospital computer system. Forty-five days after each surgical procedure, the nurse reviewer completes the patient's data entry and,

with the chief of surgery's concurrence, transmits the data to the national data coordinating center; workload and laboratory data are automatically captured and transmitted from the VA electronic data systems.

Data received at the national center are edited for missing or out-of-range values and data inconsistencies. Cleaned data are then entered into the NSQIP master file. Logistic regression analysis is used to develop the models predicting probability of death or complication (within 30 days of the major surgery in or out of hospital). Probabilities are calculated for each patient based on that patient's preoperative risk factors. Within each subspecialty and for all surgical procedures, probabilities are then summed for each hospital providing the "expected" number of events based on the patient's preoperative risks, allowing calculation of observed/expected (O/E) event ratios. Statistically significant low (O/E < 1) or high (O/E > 1) outliers are then identified to support continuous quality improvement activities. An annual report is generated and distributed to the chief of surgery, the nurse reviewers, each hospital's director and chief of staff, and the regional chief medical officer. In the report, each hospital is identified by a specific code known only to the providers, the managers at that hospital, and the regional chief medical officer. In addition, tables of the observed and expected outcomes and O/E ratios at each medical center are reviewed annually by the NSQIP Executive Committee, which forwards recommendations regarding specific hospitals in accordance with established guidelines. The latter are disseminated with the annual report.

The NSQIP has garnered the acceptance of VA surgeons and health care managers, and has provided annual outcome reports that have contributed to improving the standard of surgical care: Since 1991, unadjusted 30-day mortality and morbidity rates for major noncardiac surgery within the VA have decreased from 3.2% and 17.4% to 2.3% and 9.9%, respectively [55,57].

The program's obvious success within the VA has generated substantial interest in its application in non-VA institutions. In 1999 a preliminary attempt was made to implement the NSQIP's case identification and data collection methodology in three non-VA hospitals [58]. In this "alpha" trial, infrastructure needed to support data abstraction and reporting in the non-VA hospitals was established. This successful trial identified significant bivariate relationships between at least two thirds of the NSQIP preoperative risk variables and 30 day mortality and morbidity in the non-VA hospitals. In addition, the VA risk-adjustment models afforded high predictability when applied to the non-VA data.

The success of this trial not only demonstrated the feasibility of deploying the NSQIP in these centers, but also afforded preliminary data supporting the trial's expansion into 14 additional non-VA hospitals [58]. This expanded trial, which was supported by an AHRQ grant and coordinated by the ACS, was completed in 2004. Results from this trial are just being released, but once again demonstrate the applicability of the NSQIP methodology within the non-federal system, as well as the ability of the process to effect improvement in surgical outcomes [56,59]. Of note, many of the sub-studies generated by this research effort have finally allowed comparisons of VA and private sector risk-adjusted outcomes [60–63], at long last beginning to meet the original Congressional mandate that lead to the creation of the NSQIP [54].

This positive experience has led to the adoption and national dissemination of the NSQIP into the private sector by the American College of Surgeons (ACS-NSQIP), powered by what is now known as the www.acsnsqip. org Web site. The latter provides a mechanism by which data can be securely submitted via the Internet from hospitals with disparate medical record systems [58]. Over the past 3 years, this site has been continually enhanced; recently, a new interface was added to automatically transfer data from hospital systems directly to the central Web server. In addition, although the program initially targeted only general and vascular surgery, the ACS-NSQIP is finalizing methodology that will allow all participating sites to submit cases from multiple surgical subspecialties [64]. Other productivity tools are under development to facilitate not only the mechanics of data collection, but also to support process management and decision-making.

To date, over 150 hospitals have joined the ACS-NSQIP [65]. The program provides an ever-growing source of reliable clinical data from which to launch national surgical quality improvement initiatives and establish national surgical policy. Indeed, one such initiative, seeking to link SSI process measures with risk-adjusted outcomes and define SSI best practices, has recently begun. In another interesting development, the ACS-NSQIP has provided the critical component used to establish a unique collaboration between payers and surgical care providers [66]. In this project, termed the Michigan Surgical Quality Collaborative, Blue Cross Blue Shield of Michigan is funding statewide surgical registries and quality improvement programs in cardiac, bariatric, and other areas of general and vascular surgery [66]. Hospitals and physician groups are compensated for their data collection efforts and participation in the quality improvement activities, regardless of their individual outcomes. Success will be defined primarily by improvement in statewide surgical outcomes. Thus, as the ACS-NSQIP continues to expand and pursue its ambitious strategic plan [56], it could well serve as an outcomes measurement platform in support of a national surgical quality improvement initiative.

Summary

Given the complex interplay of structure, process, and outcomes, assessment of surgical quality presents a daunting task. As noted above, we must firmly establish the links between these elements to validate current as well as future metrics, while engendering "buy-in" on the part of surgeons.

Clearly, new paradigms and flexible approaches will need to be considered. Birkmeyer and colleagues [6] have suggested an intriguing strategy for design of procedure level monitors, based on the procedure's baseline risk and frequency. Others have suggested that any national surgical quality program should be implemented in phases, so as to support continuous quality improvement while allowing further development, refinement, and validation of newly designed measures [7]. Because surgical care providers will ultimately be held accountable for these metrics, it is vital that they be involved in their design and implementation.

We must also remember that there are many other components of surgical quality currently not well-addressed by the "traditional" metrics of mortality, morbidity, length of stay, and so forth. Patient-centered outcomes such as functional status, quality of life, and satisfaction, as well as the appropriateness of care, must be added to the list of factors comprising surgical quality. It is only by expanding our involvement in the ongoing march of quality programs that we might ultimately achieve the "holy grail of surgical quality improvement" [67].

References

[1] Committee on Quality of Health Care in America, Institute of Medicine. To err is human: building a safer health system. Washington, DC: National Academy Press; 2000.

[2] Committee on Quality of Health Care in America, Institute of Medicine. Crossing the quality chasm: a new health system for the 21st century. Washington, DC: National Academy Press; 2001.

[3] Deas TM Jr. Health care value-based purchasing. Gastrointest Endosc Clin N Am 2006;16: 643–56.

[4] Donabedian A. The quality of care. How can it be assessed? JAMA 1988;260:1743–8.

[5] Donabedian A. Evaluating the quality of medical care. 1966. Milbank Q 2005;83:691–729.

[6] Birkmeyer JD, Dimick JB, Birkmeyer NJ. Measuring the quality of surgical care: structure, process, or outcomes? J Am Coll Surg 2004;198:626–32.

[7] Jones RS, Brown C, Opelka F. Surgeon compensation: "pay for performance," the American College of Surgeons National Surgical Quality Improvement Program, the Surgical Care Improvement Program, and other considerations. Surgery 2005;138:829–36.

[8] Van Colt H. Human errors: their causes and reductions. In: Bogner MS, editor. Human error in medicine. Hillsdale (NJ): Lawrence Erlbaum Associates, Inc.; 1994. p. 53–65.

[9] Rhodes RS. Patient safety in surgical care: a systems approach in ASC surgery: principles and practice of surgery. Available at: www.medscape.com/viewarticle/456211, 2003. Accessed May 5, 2007.

[10] Edmondson AC. Learning from failure in healthcare: frequent opportunities, pervasive barriers. Qual Saf Health Care 2004;13(Suppl 2):ii3–9.

[11] Daley J, Forbes MG, Young GJ, et al. Validating risk-adjusted surgical outcomes: site visit assessment of process and structure. National VA Surgical Risk study. J Am Coll Surg 1997; 185:341–51.

[12] Hannan EL, Kilburn H Jr, O'Donnell JF, et al. Adult open heart surgery in New York State. An analysis of risk factors and hospital mortality rates. JAMA 1990;264:2768–74.

[13] O'Connor GT, Plume SK, Olmstead EM, et al. A regional intervention to improve the hospital mortality associated with coronary artery bypass graft surgery. The Northern New England Cardiovascular Disease Study Group. JAMA 1996;275:841–6.

[14] Knaus W, Draper E, Wagner D, et al. An evaluation of outcome from intensive care in major medical centers. Ann Int Med 1986;104:410–8.

[15] Frommater D, Marshall D, Halford G, et al. How a three-campus heart service line improves clinical processes and outcomes. Jt Comm J Qual Improv 1995;21:263–76.

[16] Keller RB, Griffin E, Schneiter EJ, et al. Searching for quality in medical care: The Maine Medical Assessment Foundation. J Ambul Care Manage 2002;25:63–79.

[17] Birkmeyer JD, Siewers AE, Finlayson EV, et al. Hospital volume and surgical mortality in the United States. N Engl J Med 2002;346:1128–37.

[18] Birkmeyer JD, Dimick JB. Potential benefits of the new Leapfrog standards: effect of process and outcomes measures. Surgery 2004;135:569–75.

[19] Sowden AJ, Sheldon TA. Does volume really affect outcome? Lessons from the evidence. J Health Serv Res Policy 1998;3:187–90.

[20] Betensky RA, Christian CK, Gustafson ML, et al. Hospital volume versus outcome: an unusual example of bivariate association. Biometrics 2006;62:598–604.

[21] Christian CK, Gustafson ML, Betensky RA, et al. The Leapfrog volume criteria may fall short in identifying high-quality surgical centers. Ann Surg 2003;238:447–55.

[22] Christian CK, Gustafson ML, Betensky RA, et al. The volume-outcome relationship: don't believe everything you see. World J Surg 2005;29:1241–4.

[23] Khuri SF, Daley J, Henderson W, et al. Relation of surgical volume to outcome in eight common operations: results from the VA National Surgical Quality Improvement Program. Ann Surg 1999;230:414–29.

[24] Khuri SF, Henderson WG. The case against volume as a measure of quality of surgical care. World J Surg 2005;29:1222–9.

[25] Neumayer LA, Gawande AA, Wang J, et al. Proficiency of surgeons in inguinal hernia repair: effect of experience and age. Ann Surg 2005;242:344–8.

[26] Birkmeyer JD, Dimick JB, Staiger DO. Operative mortality and procedure volume as predictors of subsequent hospital performance. Ann Surg 2006;243:411–7.

[27] Dimick JB, Birkmeyer JD, Upchurch GR Jr. Measuring surgical quality: what's the role of provider volume? World J Surg 2005;29:1217–21.

[28] Itani KM, Wilson SE, Awad SS, et al. Polyethylene glycol versus sodium phosphate mechanical bowel preparation in elective colorectal surgery. Am J Surg 2007;193:190–4.

[29] Bradley EH, Herrin J, Elbel B, et al. Hospital quality for acute myocardial infarction: correlation among process measures and relationship with short-term mortality. JAMA 2006; 296:72–8.

[30] Bratzler DW, Houck PM. Antimicrobial prophylaxis for surgery: an advisory statement from the National Surgical Infection Prevention Project. Clin Infect Dis 2004;38: 1706–15.

[31] Bratzler DW, Houck PM. Antimicrobial prophylaxis for surgery: an advisory statement from the National Surgical Infection Prevention Project. Am J Surg 2005;189:395–404.

[32] Dellinger EP, Hausmann SM, Bratzler DW, et al. Hospitals collaborate to decrease surgical site infections. Am J Surg 2005;190:9–15.

[33] SCIP Project Information. Available at: www.medqic/scip. Accessed May 5, 2007.

[34] Devereaux PJ, Beattie WS, Choi PT, et al. How strong is the evidence for the use of perioperative beta blockers in non-cardiac surgery? Systematic review and meta-analysis of randomised controlled trials. BMJ 2005;331:313–21.

[35] S.1932. Deficit Reduction Act of 2005. Congressional Budget Office (CBO). Available at: http://www.cbo.gov/ftpdocs/70xx/doc7028/s1932conf.pdf. Accessed May 5, 2007.

[36] Kahn CN III, Ault T, Isenstein H, et al. Snapshot of hospital quality reporting and pay-for-performance under Medicare. Health Aff 2006;25:148–62.

[37] Iezzoni LI. Assessing quality using administrative data. Ann Intern Med 1997;127:666–74.

[38] Main DS, Henderson WG, Pratte K, et al. Relationship of process and structures of care in general surgery to post-operative outcomes: a descriptive analysis. J Am Coll Surg 2007;204:1157–65.

[39] Main DS, Cavender TA, Nowels CT, et al. Relationship of process and structures of care in general surgery to postoperative outcomes: a qualitative study. J Am Coll Surg 2007;204: 1147–56.

[40] Iezzoni LI. An introduction to risk adjustment. Am J Med Qual 1996;11:S8–11.

[41] Iezzoni LI. The risks of risk adjustment. JAMA 1997;278:1600–7.

[42] Iezzoni LI, Ash AS, Shwartz M, et al. Predicting who dies depends on how severity is measured: implications for evaluating patient outcomes. Ann Intern Med 1995;123: 763–70.

[43] Atherly A, Fink AS, Campbell DC, et al. Evaluating alternative risk-adjustment strategies for surgery. Am J Surg 2004;188:566–70.

[44] McClure W. Competition and the pursuit of quality: a conversation with Walter McClure. Interview by John K. Iglehart. Health Aff (Millwood) 1988;7:79–90.

[45] Rosenthal GE, Harper DL. Cleveland Health Quality Choice: a model for collaborative community-based outcomes assessment. Jt Comm J Qual Improv 1994;20:425–42.

[46] Daley J, Khuri SF, Henderson W, et al. Risk adjustment of the postoperative morbidity rate for the comparative assessment of the quality of surgical care: results of the National Veterans Affairs Surgical Risk Study. J Am Coll Surg 1997;185:328–40.

[47] Khuri SF, Daley J, Henderson W, et al. The National Veterans Administration Surgical Risk Study: risk adjustment for the comparative assessment of the quality of surgical care. J Am Coll Surg 1995;180:519–31.

[48] Khuri SF, Daley J, Henderson W, et al. Risk adjustment of the postoperative mortality rate for the comparative assessment of the quality of surgical care: results of the National Veterans Affairs Surgical Risk Study. J Am Coll Surg 1997;185:315–27.

[49] Khuri SF, Daley J, Henderson W, et al. The Department of Veterans Affairs' NSQIP: the first national, validated, outcome-based, risk-adjusted, and peer-controlled program for the measurement and enhancement of the quality of surgical care. National VA Surgical Quality Improvement Program. Ann Surg 1998;228:491–507.

[50] Rosen HM, Green BA. The HCFA excess mortality lists: a methodological critique. Hosp Health Serv Adm 1987;32:119–27.

[51] Dubois RW. Inherent limitations of hospital death rates to assess quality. Int J Technol Assess Health Care 1990;6:220–8.

[52] US General Accounting Office Health EaHSD. Employers and individual consumers want additional information on quality GAO/HEHS-95-201. . Washington, DC: U.S. General Accounting Office; 1995.

[53] Freeman JL, Fetter RB, Park H, et al. Diagnosis-related group refinement with diagnosis- and procedure-specific comorbidities and complications. Med Care 1995;33:806–27.

[54] Veterans Administration Health-Care Amendments of 1985. II: Health Care Administration, 204. 2006. 99 STAT 941. 12-3-1985.

[55] Khuri SF, Daley J, Henderson WG. The comparative assessment and improvement of quality of surgical care in the Department of Veterans Affairs. Arch Surg 2002;137:20–7.

[56] Khuri SF. The NSQIP: a new frontier in surgery. Surgery 2005;138:837–43.

[57] Khuri SF. Quality, advocacy, healthcare policy, and the surgeon. Ann Thorac Surg 2002;74: 641–9.

[58] Fink AS, Campbell DA Jr, Mentzer RM Jr, et al. The National Surgical Quality Improvement Program in non-Veterans Administration hospitals: initial demonstration of feasibility. Ann Surg 2002;236:344–53.

[59] Khuri S, Henderson W, Daley J, et al. Successful implementation of the Department of Veterans Affairs' NSQIP in the private sector: the patient safety in surgery study. Submitted to NEJM.

[60] Fink AS, Hutter MM, Campbell DA Jr, et al. Comparison of risk-adjusted 30-day post-operative mortality and morbidity in Department of Veterans Affairs hospitals and selected university medical centers: general surgical operations in females. J Am Coll Surg 2007; 204:1127–36.

[61] Henderson W, Khuri S, Mosca C, et al. Comparison of risk-adjusted 30-day post-operative mortality and morbidity in Department of Veterans Affairs hospitals and selected university medical centers: general surgical operations in males. J Am Coll Surg 2007;204:1103–14.

[62] Hutter MM, Lancaster RT, Henderson WG, et al. Comparison of risk-adjusted 30-day post-operative mortality and morbidity in Department of Veterans Affairs hospitals and selected university medical centers: vascular operations in men. J Am Coll Surg 2007;204:1115–26.

[63] Johnson RG, Wittgen CM, Hutter MM, et al. Comparison of risk-adjusted 30-day postoperative mortality and morbidity in Department of Veteran Affairs hospitals and selected university medical centers: vascular surgical operations in women. J Am Coll Surg 2007;204: 1137–46.

[64] American College of Surgeons National Surgical Quality Improvement Program. Available at: https://acsnsqip.org/main/about_news.asp. Accessed May 6, 2007.

[65] American College of Surgeons National Surgical Quality Improvement Program. Available at: https://acsnsqip.org/main/about_sites.asp. Accessed May 6, 2007.

[66] Birkmeyer NJ, Share D, Campbell DA Jr, et al. Partnering with payers to improve surgical quality: the Michigan plan. Surgery 2005;138:815–20.

[67] Rogers SO Jr. The holy grail of surgical quality improvement: process measures or risk-adjusted outcomes? Am Surg 2006;72:1046–50.

ELSEVIER
SAUNDERS

SURGICAL
CLINICS OF
NORTH AMERICA

Surg Clin N Am 87 (2007) 853–866

Safe Introduction of New Procedures and Emerging Technologies in Surgery: Education, Credentialing, and Privileging

Ajit K. Sachdeva, MD, FRCSC, FACS*,
Thomas R. Russell, MD, FACS

American College of Surgeons, 633 N. Saint Clair Street, Chicago, IL 60611-3211, USA

Advances in science and technology have led to modifications in established procedures and introduction of entirely new procedures and technologies in surgery. Such advances continue to impact surgical practice. Patients benefit from the advances through access to more safe and effective treatment modalities or enhancement of quality of life. Unless concrete steps are taken to ensure safe introduction of a new procedure or technology into surgical practice, however, patients may be placed at undue risk.

A surgeon's decision to adopt a new procedure or technology may be influenced by numerous intrinsic and extrinsic factors. These include the desire to provide the best care to patients, the lure of the procedure or technology, the drive to remain competitive, or pressures from health care systems, industry, and even the patients themselves [1]. Self-regulation by surgeons, individually and collectively as a profession, remains key to ensuring patient safety. This requires the highest levels of professionalism. Unless the surgical profession regulates itself diligently and demonstrates transparency in this process, external regulatory bodies and the government may get involved [2].

Introduction of new procedures such as laparoscopic cholecystectomy, sentinel lymph node biopsy, carotid stent placement, and total mesorectal excision into surgical practice has demonstrated the need for several key

---

This article originally published in the *Surgical Oncology Clinics of North America*, January 2007. pp. 101–14.

The opinions expressed in this article are those of the authors and do not necessarily reflect the official positions of the American College of Surgeons.

* Corresponding author.

E-mail address: asachdeva@facs.org (A.K. Sachdeva).

doi:10.1016/j.suc.2007.06.006

steps. These include objectively assessing the new procedure or emerging technology using evidence-based information, offering educational interventions to help surgeons acquire the requisite knowledge and skills, supporting safe and effective introduction of new surgical modalities into practice, monitoring of outcomes, credentialing and privileging of surgeons and surgical teams, and educating patients.

Assessment of a new procedure or emerging technology

New procedures and emerging technologies need to be identified and evaluated through a process of ongoing and systematic horizon scanning. A thorough analysis of the risks versus benefits is essential. The evaluation should focus not only on assessing the safety and efficacy of the new modality in controlled settings but also on how the modality will be used in practice [3]. Introduction of a new procedure or an emerging technology should be timed carefully and strike a balance between waiting for sufficient data to support its use and the health care needs of patients while data are being collected. Late introduction of a new modality may deprive the patients of adequate or state-of-the-art care. The surgical profession must intervene promptly to modify or discontinue a new procedure or technology if it is found to be unsafe or ineffective before it causes widespread harm. Yet, sufficient time is needed to permit appropriate adoption and use of the new modality in practice.

Evidence-based information relating to safety and efficacy of a new procedure or emerging technology may be obtained through national or regional sources. Professional surgical organizations such as the American College of Surgeons (ACS) are working on establishing systems for ongoing collection, analysis, and dissemination of evidence-based information. Such systems should involve evaluation of available evidence relating to the new procedure or emerging technology by experts in the field and provision of guidance to surgeons regarding safe adoption of the new modality in practice. The Internet offers a convenient means for disseminating and regularly updating this information.

Information from national or regional sources must be evaluated at the local level to make decisions regarding introduction of a new modality within an institution. This permits assessment of the evidence within the context of specific local needs. The process should take into consideration the following:

- The patients served
- The educational interventions that will be required to address the learning needs of surgeons, members of the surgical team, and patients
- The systems and infrastructure necessary to deliver safe and effective care
- The fiscal impact

While using an evidence-based approach, the reviewers must recognize its limitations. Randomized controlled clinical trials are difficult to implement in surgery, and variations in the performance of a procedure or use of a technology can influence outcomes [3]. A new procedure or emerging technology that is supported by evidence regarding its safety and efficacy should be handled differently as compared with a procedure or technology that has not yet proven to be safe and efficacious. In the latter situation, the new modality must be introduced only within the framework of a clinical trial following approval by the local institutional review board. Evaluation of the safety and effectiveness of a new procedure or technology should continue following its introduction into surgical practice. The evaluation of any new modality must include all parties involved with the introduction of the modality, such as surgeons, members of the surgical team, other health care professionals, and administrators.

The surgeon should assess his or her practice needs and determine whether a new procedure or an emerging technology should be adopted in the surgeon's practice. This process needs to involve review of evidence regarding the new modality and a systematic gap analysis of the surgeon's practice. Such gap analyses should be based on reviewing the surgeon's outcomes data and benchmarking these with national, regional, or local standards. Once the surgeon has made the decision to pursue adoption of a new procedure or emerging technology in his or her practice, the next step is participation in an appropriate educational program.

Educational interventions

Background

Education plays a critical role in the safe introduction of a new procedure or technology into surgical practice. The Center for Devices and Radiological Health of the US Food and Drug Administration (FDA) evaluates new devices and technologies and approves their use in practice. The training programs proposed for the devices and technologies are reviewed before granting approval. Also, the device manufacturing companies often are asked to include assessment of the training program in the postapproval study of a new device and to modify the training program based on results of this assessment (Kenneth J. Cavanaugh, Jr, personal communication, 2006). The FDA, however, does not dictate the content of the training program or the specific educational methods that should be used. The responsibility for educating surgeons and members of the surgical team rests primarily with professional organizations such as surgical specialty societies, and with local institutions. These entities need to assume the responsibility for designing and implementing state-of-the-art educational programs to help surgeons and surgical teams acquire the requisite knowledge and skills to provide optimum care.

Educational principles and methods

A disease-based approach rather than a technology-driven approach should be used in designing and implementing educational interventions to address knowledge and skills in new procedures and emerging technologies. Educational programs should support not just the acquisition of knowledge and skills and demonstration of competence, but also changes in surgeons' practices to impact surgical outcomes. A complete educational model that includes structured teaching and learning, verification of knowledge and skills, postcourse preceptoring or proctoring, and monitoring of outcomes is needed to achieve the best results. Because of the different educational needs of individual surgeons, prerequisite knowledge and skills for each course need to be defined specifically. Interactive and contextually relevant educational interventions that are based on specific needs assessments are more effective in changing practices, as compared with passive learning experiences that are not linked to the specific needs of individual learners. Also, sequenced and multifaceted interventions that involve multiple formats and are complemented by enabling and reinforcing strategies, such as educational materials, reminders, and feedback, are important in changing practices and impacting patient outcomes [4,5]. While designing and implementing educational programs, the learning needs of the entire surgical team and various aspects of the systems in which the new procedure or emerging technology will be introduced need to be addressed to ensure optimum outcomes.

Short courses in new procedures and emerging technologies, often offered over weekends, have been used frequently to teach surgeons new skills. Such courses in isolation are not sufficient to promote safe patient care. A higher complication rate has been reported for surgeons who participated in an isolated laparoscopic surgery course without additional training [6]. Other predictors of complications following this training included attending the training course alone, working in a solo practice setting, and operating with variable assistants.

When designing an educational program, attempts should be made to standardize the performance of a procedure or use of a technology. Each procedure should be broken down into its component tasks through a detailed task analysis, and then the skills need to be practiced, ideally in simulated laboratory settings, until the desired level of proficiency is achieved before working with patients in real environments. Various bench models, simulations, simulators, and virtual tools are available to assist in teaching, learning, and assessing surgical skills. Low-fidelity bench models may be used to address basic surgical skills [7]. Use of such low-fidelity bench models can simplify implementation of educational interventions. Higher-fidelity simulations may be reserved for teaching, learning, and assessing complex surgical skills, judgment, situational awareness, and teamwork. Skills acquired in virtual environments have been shown to transfer to the operating room [8]. Thus, training in laboratory settings before working with patients should be beneficial. Once new knowledge and skills are acquired, development of expertise requires deliberate practice coupled with specific feedback [9]. Ongoing improvement in performance results from establishing educational goals that exceed current levels of performance. Learner motivation and accurate self-assessment also play an important role in the development of expertise [10].

Objective assessment of new knowledge and skills should be conducted using valid and reliable tools. A model for objective and structured assessment of technical skills in laboratory settings has been described [11]. This has been implemented successfully at several institutions to assess the technical skills of residents, and should also be useful in assessing the skills of practicing surgeons. Assessment of surgical skills in the operating room is generally subjective. Such assessments, however, may be enhanced through structured methods that involve use of global assessment scales. The validity and reliability of a global assessment tool for the intraoperative assessment of laparoscopic skills has been demonstrated [12].

The three major variables that influence acquisition of a surgical skill are the complexity of the skill, the innate ability of the surgeon, and the training of the surgeon [10]. The individual learning curve of the surgeon must be considered during the educational intervention. The learning curve is a graphic representation of the relationship between experience with the procedure or technology, which may be reflected by the numbers of cases performed, and an outcome variable such as complications or operating time [13]. Learning curves vary with the skill of the surgeon and the complexity of the task, and these may be impacted by the surgical findings, such as pathology and anatomic variations. During the early stages of experience with a new modality, the learning curve is steep, and the curve becomes flatter with more experience. The risk to the patient is greatest during the steep portion of the learning curve; thus, special safeguards are needed to minimize risk. An effective strategy is to use preceptors to help surgeon learners during the steep part of the learning curve.

Preceptoring and proctoring

Preceptoring can be implemented using numerous different models. The preceptor may work with the surgeon learner at the learner's institution; the surgeon learner may bring the patient to the preceptor's institution; or the preceptoring may be conducted through a mini-fellowship [10]. Each model has advantages and disadvantages. The principal role of a preceptor is to serve as a teacher and coach to help the learner acquire new knowledge and skills. The preceptor assesses and verifies the learner's knowledge and skills using valid and reliable methods and provides feedback to the learner. Generally, preceptors are experts in performing the new procedure or using the emerging technology and often scrub in with surgeon learners to guide the learners as teaching assistants [14]. The preceptor retains the overall responsibility for the patient's care in the operating room and is able to readily take over the operation if the situation demands. This helps in ensuring patient safety. Although preceptoring can be very useful in helping surgeons acquire new surgical knowledge and skills, logistics such as legal risk and time constraints discourage experienced surgeons from serving as preceptors.

Performance of surgeon learners also may be observed and assessed by proctors. The involvement of proctors during the early stages of performing a new procedure or using a new technology has been found to be helpful [14]. The principal role of a proctor is to assess and verify the knowledge and skills of the surgeon learner using valid and reliable methods. Proctors serve as observers and generally do not teach surgeon learners. They may provide feedback to learners, but that is not their main function. The proctor is responsible for reporting the results of the assessment of the surgeon learner to the Chief of Surgery or the credentialing committee of the institution. The logistical issues associated with proctoring are less complex than those associated with preceptoring, and the legal risk is less. The principal differences between the roles and responsibilities of a preceptor and proctor are listed in the Box 1.

Several creative strategies have been used to address the complexities associated with the implementation of preceptoring and proctoring. A surgeon may undergo an appropriate educational experience and then serve as a preceptor for other surgeons within a department [2]. If a preceptor is not readily available, reciprocal proctoring may be helpful [14]. This involves two surgeons completing a course and then performing their first several procedures together, alternately serving as operating surgeon and first assistant. Each surgeon reports on the other's performance to the Chief of Surgery or the institutional credentialing committee. Another innovative educational approach involves telepreceptoring and teleproctoring [15,16]. Remote teaching and assessment are conducted by experts using technology support. Image-based procedures lend themselves well to telepreceptoring and teleproctoring, and telepreceptoring has been demonstrated to be effective within the context of laparoscopic surgery [16]. As course faculty members are trained in innovative educational techniques involving telepreceptoring and teleproctoring, and technology develops further, these methods are likely to play a more prominent role in the education of surgeons. Regardless of the mechanism used for preceptoring or proctoring, institutions need to develop and implement appropriate strategies to ensure safe introduction of new procedures and emerging technologies.

Transition to independent practice and monitoring of outcomes

As surgeons begin to perform a new procedure or use a new technology independently, appropriate case mix and careful patient selection are

---

Box 1. Principal differences between the roles and responsibilities of a preceptor and proctor

Preceptor
- Principal role is to help the surgeon learner acquire new surgical knowledge and skills during the steep portion of the learning curve.
- Assesses and verifies the knowledge and skills of the surgeon learner to ensure achievement of learning objectives
- Always provides feedback to the learner
- Must be an expert in the performance of the new procedure or use of the new technology; such expertise is necessary for effective preceptoring
- Generally assists in the operation and is readily available to take charge if the need arises
- Associated with greater legal risk
- Logistics more complex

Proctor
- Principal role is to assess the knowledge and skills of the surgeon learner during the steep portion of the learning curve
- Assesses and verifies the knowledge and skills of the surgeon learner to report the results to the Chief of Surgery or the institutional credentialing committee
- May provide feedback to the learner
- Does not always need to be an expert in the performance of a new procedure or use of a new technology; such expertise is desirable but not always necessary for effective proctoring
- Generally serves as an observer
- Associated with lesser legal risk
- Logistics less complex

---

necessary. A few harder cases may be selected following the initial experience to enhance skills and promote development of expertise. Several national organizations have suggested minimum numbers of cases that should be performed to ensure proficiency. Although sufficient case volume is necessary for acquisition and maintenance of surgical skills, consideration of the numbers of cases alone is inadequate because of the other variables involved. These include the abilities and skill of the learner, specifics of the patient's problem, complexity of the task involved, skills of the other team members, and institutional systems. In addition, the quality of the educational experience directly impacts the surgeon's knowledge and skills, and such experiences are not always consistent. Consideration of numbers of cases alone may result in establishment of higher standards than needed to ensure proficiency, or worse, inadequate standards that would compromise patient safety.

The cycle of practice-based learning and improvement (PBLI) provides a useful framework to link education in new procedures and emerging technologies with the delivery of safe and optimum patient care. Steps of the PBLI Cycle are (1) identifying areas for improvement, (2) engaging in learning, (3) applying new knowledge and skills to practice, and (4) checking for improvement [17]. Monitoring of a surgeon's experience should include analysis and evaluation of data on indications, patient selection, and outcomes. Ideally, prospective and risk-adjusted methods should be used to assess surgical outcomes. Monitoring of outcomes should be linked closely with the ongoing quality assurance activities of an institution. Such assessments can provide valuable information, not just on the skills of the individual surgeon, but also on issues relating to the safety and effectiveness of the new procedure or technology, problems with education of the surgical team, and adequacy of systems in which the new modality is being introduced. Ongoing assessment of outcomes is necessary once the modality has been adopted in surgical practice. The surgeon's practice needs to be monitored closely for a sufficient period of time, because initial acceptable levels of performance might be followed by deterioration in the surgeon's outcomes because of poor patient selection or overconfidence. If ongoing monitoring indicates a problem with a surgeon's skills, remediation through retraining and additional preceptoring may become necessary. Important lessons learned through the monitoring process need to be shared with other surgeons to benefit the broad cross-section of patients. National outcomes databases should be created to collect information on the results of introduction of a new procedure or emerging technology in practice and to benchmark an individual surgeon's outcomes data or an institution's experience with others across the country.

Regional support for educational programs

Regional support for education in new procedures and emerging technologies is essential to enhance access to educational opportunities. This may be offered through the establishment of a national network of skills or education centers [13,18,19]. Such centers can play a pivotal role in offering state-of-the-art educational programs that include structured teaching and learning, objective and reliable verification of knowledge and skills, and postcourse preceptoring or proctoring. The centers also may create supportive regional learning communities to enhance the surgical care delivered regionally. The ACS recently launched a program for accreditation of education institutes that is being implemented under the aegis of the ACS Division of Education [19]. The ACS-accredited Education Institutes will offer a range of educational programs to address knowledge and skills in new procedures and emerging technologies. Certain educational programs will be developed by the ACS, whereas others will be developed locally. The institutes will be encouraged to consider offering educational programs to various learners, including surgeons, members of the surgical team, and patients, and to reach out locally and regionally to address the needs of these learner groups. Some institutes would serve as national demonstration sites for innovative educational approaches involving the use of certain new procedures and emerging technologies.

Accreditation is being offered to the institutes by the ACS at two levels: Level I, Comprehensive; and Level II, Basic. Three standards are being used to accredit the institutions: Learners, Curriculum, and Technical Support and Resources. Institutes accredited at Level I are expected to offer a complete range of educational programs to address complex knowledge and skills using state-of-the-art simulations, simulators, and cutting-edge technologies. They also may pursue preceptoring and proctoring, faculty development, and research. Institutes accredited at Level II are expected to offer educational programs to address basic knowledge and skills. Simple simulations and bench models may be used by these institutes to achieve the desired educational outcomes.

Focus on the learners

Although efforts of national organizations and local institutions are key to offering surgeons state-of-the-art educational opportunities, surgeons themselves need to take charge of their education and professional development. Surgeons should seek specific educational programs based on their learning needs and commit sufficient time to participate in these programs. They should be willing to participate in a complete educational experience that includes postcourse preceptoring or proctoring and monitoring of outcomes. This may not be easy because of the practical difficulties associated with busy practices. Easy access to educational opportunities offered regionally and availability of selected educational content on the Internet should facilitate participation and make the process less burdensome. Also, support from the surgeon's department and institution is essential to facilitate the surgeon's participation in a complete educational program.

As new procedures or technologies are introduced into surgical practice, the learning needs of surgical residents also should be addressed. The logistics of teaching new skills to residents are comparatively simple relative to the logistics involved with teaching new skills to practicing surgeons. This is because of the availability of structured educational opportunities within residency programs. Also, as new procedures and technologies are introduced into surgical practice and surgeons are trained in these new modalities, residents will be exposed to the modalities during their training and benefit from teaching provided by the surgical faculty. Special national courses for residents may supplement local efforts of the faculty.

Safe introduction of new procedures and emerging technologies into surgical practice requires education of the entire surgical team. Specific educational needs of each team member must be addressed with the same rigor as that used for educating surgeons and surgical residents. Collaborative teamwork involving various professionals is essential to ensure safety and optimum outcomes. This too should be addressed through educational interventions.

The special role of patients in the safe introduction of new procedures or technologies requires special attention. Education of patients is important for them to participate in their care as informed and knowledgeable partners. Educational efforts should result in patients being informed sufficiently about the risks and benefits of a new procedure or technology while making decisions relating to their care. Such decisions should be made in close collaboration with the surgeon. Educated patients are less likely to demand the use of a new modality before establishment of its safety and efficacy. Also, patients educated in the various aspects of their perioperative care are more likely to take better care of themselves, identify adverse events early, and bring important issues to the attention of the surgeon and other members of the surgical team in a timely fashion. This should help to promote patient safety, enhance surgical outcomes, and aid in the recovery of the patient following the surgical procedure.

Special considerations

Introduction of a new procedure or an emerging technology involves consideration of special nuances relating to the new modality. The complete spectrum of cognitive, clinical, and technical skills needs to be addressed. The learner must acquire the requisite skills to provide optimum patient care before, during, and following the intervention. The value of interdisciplinary collaboration has been demonstrated within the context of new procedures such as sentinel lymph node biopsy, carotid stent placement, and total mesorectal excision [20–28].

The special aspects of training surgeons to perform sentinel lymph node biopsy have been described by several authors [20–22]. One such nuance involves assessment of the learner. Performance of sentinel lymph node biopsy followed by completion axillary lymph node dissection has been used to assess the identification rate and accuracy of sentinel lymph node biopsy. This offers an accurate yardstick for proficiency assessment. Collaboration across the interdisciplinary team of trained surgeons, nuclear medicine specialists, and pathologists is necessary to achieve optimum outcomes.

Introduction of carotid stent placement has revealed several unique challenges [23,24]. Education in carotid stent placement has demonstrated blurring of traditional specialty-specific lines and has underscored the need for disease-based educational approaches. Because physicians from numerous different specialties, including vascular surgery, interventional cardiology, and interventional radiology, may perform this procedure, the physicians from these specialties enter educational programs with different levels of baseline knowledge and skills. Thus, the specific prerequisites for participation in educational programs must be defined and the educational experience tailored to meet the needs of the specialty group and the individual surgeon or physician. A broad range of cognitive skills, including comprehensive knowledge of cardiovascular disease, diagnostic approaches, and therapeutic options, is needed to provide optimum care. Also, the technical skills education relating to carotid stent placement requires baseline expertise in catheter-based interventions. Because of the high risk of stroke, sufficient experience on a simulator and achievement of proficiency in laboratory settings before work with patients are recommended highly.

Introduction of another new procedure, total mesorectal excision, has highlighted the need for educational interventions that focus on standardized techniques to ensure optimum outcomes [25–28]. Once again, the training of the interdisciplinary team, including the surgeon and the pathologist, has been found to be important.

Credentialing and privileging to perform new procedures and use emerging technologies

The Joint Commission has defined standards for credentialing and privileging to promote delivery of safe and high-quality patient care [29,30]. Credentialing involves collection, verification, and assessment of information regarding the licensure of the surgeon; the surgeon's education, training, and experience; and the surgeon's current competence to perform the procedure or use the technology. Accurate documentation of education and relevant training, including the proficiency achieved, is very useful in this context. Also, letters describing the surgeon's proficiency from preceptors, proctors, qualified peers, and the department chair are helpful if they include objective, valid, and reliable information. The process of granting privileges to perform a procedure or use a new technology is based on review of the surgeon's performance and should include assessment of outcomes data relating to the specific procedure or technology. Objective evaluations from preceptors, proctors, and peers, and recommendations from the surgery department chairperson remain the cornerstone of privileging. The initial privileges may be qualified and require a period of proctoring and monitoring of outcomes.

The surgery department chairperson is responsible for ensuring the delivery of optimum patient care and patient safety and fairly evaluating a surgeon's request for specific privileges. This individual plays a key role in recommending privileges for a surgeon in his or her department. The chairperson needs to objectively review the education, training, experience, and patient care outcomes of the surgeon before making a recommendation.

The role of the surgeon in requesting privileges to perform a new procedure or use a new technology is paramount. The surgeon needs to assess his or her own education and experience and possess sufficient confidence in performing the procedure or using the technology before requesting privileges. The process of self-assessment and self-regulation needs to be built on the highest standards of professionalism that emphasize patient safety above all other interests.

Several national surgical organizations have described systems for verifying surgeons' participation in educational programs, and some have offered guidelines regarding credentialing and privileging [31–34]. The ACS has defined a five-level model for verifying and documenting surgeons' participation in educational programs and the surgeon's knowledge and skills. The five levels include verification of attendance, verification of satisfactory completion of course objectives, verification of knowledge and skills, verification of preceptorial experience, and demonstration of satisfactory patient outcomes [10]. This system is being implemented, and for the first time each didactic and skills-oriented postgraduate course offered at the 2006 ACS Clinical Congress was classified using the five verification levels.

Although national organizations may provide guidance regarding credentialing standards, granting of privileges to perform a procedure or use a technology remains the prerogative of the local institution. Each institution is responsible for selecting and retaining physicians with the requisite competence; overseeing practitioners; maintaining safe and adequate facilities and equipment; and formulating, adopting, and enforcing rules and policies to ensure delivery of quality care to the patients [35]. Neglect of these responsibilities may expose the institution to risk of liability. Each institution needs to establish a system for credentialing and privileging relating to new procedures and technologies. Although privileges must be procedure-specific, the institution should decide whether a new privilege is required for each surgical device or whether there is sufficient overlap between certain devices to grant blanket approval for the use of related devices. The institution must establish clear credentialing and privileging standards and processes, which should be applied uniformly and fairly across all practitioners. Care must be taken to not allow turf and other political issues to compromise the integrity of the credentialing and privileging process [36]. Processes for ongoing monitoring of outcomes need to be defined clearly. Each institution should be responsible for demonstrating delivery of safe and optimum patient care through ongoing collection and analysis of outcomes data.

Summary

The safe introduction of a new procedure or an emerging technology into surgical practice requires ongoing horizon scanning to identify the new modalities and to evaluate evidence to support adoption of these modalities in practice. Gap analyses conducted by individual surgeons help in defining individual learning needs. Complete educational programs that include use of structured teaching and learning methods, objective assessment of knowledge and skills, preceptoring or proctoring, and monitoring of outcomes, should help in safe introduction of a new treatment modality into practice. Education of the entire surgical team is necessary. Patients need to play an active role in informed decision making and in their perioperative care. Although national organizations have established educational standards and may provide guidelines relating to credentialing and privileging, the process of granting specific privileges to individuals remains the purview of the local institution. Credentialing and privileging must not be based exclusively on the numbers of procedures performed by the surgeon, and they should be anchored to specific performance and outcomes criteria. Attention to the aforementioned items is essential to delivering the highest quality of safe and optimum care to surgical patients.

References

[1] Gates EA. New surgical procedures: can our patients benefit while we learn? Am J Obstet Gynecol 1997;176(6):1293–9.

[2] Sequeira R, Weinbaum F, Satterfield J, et al. Credentialing physicians for new technology: the physician's learning curve must not harm the patient. Am Surg 1994;60(11):821–3.

[3] Poulin P, Donnon T, Oddone Paolucci E, et al. Module 1 workshop manual: an overview: what is health technology assessment (HTA)? In: Health technology assessment. Calgary (Canada): University of Calgary; 2005. p. 6, 25.

[4] Mazmanian PE, Davis DA. Continuing medical education and the physician as a learner: guide to the evidence. JAMA 2002;288(9):1057–60.

[5] Robertson MK, Umble KE, Cervero RM. Impact studies in continuing education for health professions: update. J Contin Educ Health Prof 2003;23:146–56.

[6] See WA, Cooper CS, Fisher RJ. Predictors of laparoscopic complications after formal training in laparoscopic surgery. JAMA 1993;270(22):2689–92.

[7] Grober ED, Hamstra SJ, Wanzel KR, et al. The educational impact of bench model fidelity on the acquisition of technical skill: the use of clinically relevant outcome measures. Ann Surg 2004;240(2):374–81.

[8] Seymour NE, Gallagher AG, Roman SA, et al. Virtual reality training improves operating room performance: results of a randomized, double-blinded study. Ann Surg 2002;236(4): 458–64.

[9] Ericsson KA. Deliberate practice and the acquisition and maintenance of expert performance in medicine and related domains. Acad Med 2004;79(10 Suppl):S70–81.

[10] Sachdeva AK. Acquiring skills in new procedures and technology: the challenge and the opportunity. Arch Surg 2005;140:387–9.

[11] Reznick R, Regehr G, MacRae H, et al. Testing technical skill via an innovative "bench station" examination. Am J Surg 1997;173:226–30.

[12] Vassiliou MC, Feldman LS, Andrew CG, et al. A global assessment tool for evaluation of intraoperative laparoscopic skills. Am J Surg 2005;190:107–13.

[13] Rogers DA, Elstein AS, Bordage G. Improving continuing medical education for surgical techniques: applying the lessons learned in the first decade of minimal access surgery. Ann Surg 2001;233(2):159–66.

[14] Ballantyne GH, Kelley WE Jr. Granting clinical privileges for telerobotic surgery. Surg Laparosc Endosc Percutan Tech 2002;12(1):17–25.

[15] Rosser JC Jr, Gabriel N, Herman B, et al. Telementoring and teleproctoring. World J Surg 2001;25(11):1438–48.

[16] Panait L, Rafiq A, Tomulescu V, et al. Telementoring versus on-site mentoring in virtual reality-based surgical training. Surg Endosc 2006;20:113–8.

[17] Sachdeva AK. The new paradigm of continuing education in surgery. Arch Surg 2005;140: 264–9.

[18] Thomas-Gibson S, Williams CB. Colonoscopy training—new approaches, old problems. Gastrointest Endosc Clin N Am 2005;15:813–27.

[19] Pellegrini CA, Sachdeva AK, Johnson KA. Accreditation of education institutes by the American College of Surgeons: a new program following an old tradition. Bull Am Coll Surg 2006;91(3):9–12.

[20] Wilke LG. Training and mentoring surgeons in lymphatic mapping. Semin Oncol 2004; 31(3):333–7.

[21] Posther KE, McCall LM, Blumencranz PW, et al. Sentinel node skills verification and surgeon performance: data from a multicenter clinical trial for early-stage breast cancer. Ann Surg 2005;242(4):593–602.

[22] Cox CE, Salud CJ, Cantor A, et al. Learning curves for breast cancer sentinel lymph node mapping based on surgical volume analysis. J Am Coll Surg 2001;193(6):593–600.

[23] Rosenfeld K, Babb JD, Cates CU, et al. SCAI/SVMB/SVS clinical competence statement on carotid stenting: training and credentialing for carotid stenting—multispecialty consensus recommendations: a report of the SCAI/SVMB/SVS Writing Committee to develop a clinical competence statement on carotid interventions. Vasc Med 2005;10:65–75.

[24] Schneider PA. Optimal training strategies for carotid stenting. Semin Vasc Surg 2005;18: 69–74.

[25] Wexner SD, Rotholtz NA. Surgeon influenced variables in resectional rectal cancer surgery. Dis Colon Rectum 2000;43(11):1606–27.

[26] Mack LA, Temple WJ. Education is the key to quality of surgery for rectal cancer. Eur J Surg Oncol 2005;31:636–44.

[27] Kapiteijn E, Putter H, van de Velde CJH, et al. Impact of the introduction and training of total mesorectal excision on recurrence and survival in rectal cancer in The Netherlands. Br J Surg 2002;89:1142–9.

[28] Kapiteijn E, van de Velde CJH. Developments and quality assurance in rectal cancer surgery. Eur J Cancer 2002;38:919–36.

[29] Comprehensive accreditation manual for hospitals: the official handbook. Oakbrook Terrace (IL): Joint Commission on Accreditation of Healthcare Organizations; 2006.

[30] Proposed revisions to the medical staff credentialing and privileging standards. Oakbrook Terrace (IL): Joint Commission on Accreditation of Healthcare Organizations; 2005.

[31] Society of American Gastrointestinal Endoscopic Surgeons (SAGES). Guidelines for granting of privileges for laparoscopic and/or thoracoscopic general surgery. Surg Endosc 1998; 12:379–80.

[32] Guidelines for institutions granting privileges utilizing laparoscopic and/or thoracoscopic techniques. Society of American Gastrointestinal and Endoscopic Surgeons (SAGES), Los Angeles (CA); 2001. Available at: http://www.sages.org/sagespublicationprint.php?doc=14. Accessed June 12, 2006.

[33] Wexner SD, Eisen GM, Simmang C. Principles of privileging and credentialing for endoscopy and colonoscopy. Surg Endosc 2002;16:367–9.

[34] Tafra L, McMasters KM, Whitworth P, et al. Credentialing issues with sentinel lymph node staging for breast cancer. Am J Surg 2000;180:268–73.

[35] Stillman BC. Hospital and health plan liability in granting privileges for endoscopy. Am J Gastroenterol 2005;100:2146–8.

[36] Schneider DB, Rapp JH. Credentialing for carotid artery stenting. Perspect Vasc Surg Endovasc Ther 2005;17(2):127–34.

ELSEVIER
SAUNDERS

SURGICAL
CLINICS OF
NORTH AMERICA

Surg Clin N Am 87 (2007) 867–881

Patient Safety and Quality in Surgery

Michael H. McCafferty, MD,
Hiram C. Polk, Jr, MD*

*Department of Surgery, Section of Colorectal Surgery, University of Louisville,
550 South Jackson Street, Louisville, Kentucky 40202, USA*

Patient safety is of fundamental concern to the practicing surgeon, yet the deficiencies of our health care system in providing the degree of safety achieved by other industries are only relatively recently appreciated. Ernest Amory Codman joined the Massachusetts General Hospital staff in 1895, became interested in improving patient outcomes, and proposed the "end result idea", which would involve patient follow-up for 1 year after hospitalization. He also advocated public disclosure of outcomes by surgeons and hospital [1]. Eventually his efforts earned him pariah status.

The American College of Surgeons has stood for patient safety since its establishment in 1913. Interestingly, it founded a hospital care standards program, which eventually became the Joint Commission on Accreditation of Healthcare Organizations (JCAHO). It also formed the Committee on Cancer and the Committee on Trauma to improve the surgical care of cancer and trauma patients [2]. Safety as a system-related concern was recognized after studies of industrial catastrophes, such as major airline accidents and the Three Mile Island nuclear reactor accident in the 1970s [3,4].

In the early 1990s, medical error resulting in patient injury or death began to be appreciated as more than rare [5]. The 1999 publication by the Institute of Medicine, *To Err is Human*, estimated that between 44,000 and 98,000 patients die annually in the United States as a direct result of medical error [6]. This prompted the recognition that safety problems were real and pervasive. In addition to safety concerns, data such as are published in *The Dartmouth Atlas of Health Care* have focused attention on the unexplained regional variations in health care in the United States [7]. As health care costs have risen, payers, insurers, and consumers are keenly aware of these issues and seek solutions. Our professional responsibility is to lead the movement toward

* Corresponding author.
E-mail address: hcpolk01@louisville.edu (H.C. Polk, Jr).

0039-6109/07/$ - see front matter © 2007 Elsevier Inc. All rights reserved.
doi:10.1016/j.suc.2007.06.001   *surgical.theclinics.com*

safer and higher quality health care for our patients, first in surgery, but also throughout our practices and institutions.

Anesthesia: a model for improving safety

Our colleagues in anesthesia are leaders in medicine in recognizing safety issues from within, objectively studying the problems, implementing changes, and demonstrating improved outcomes. Lanier has succinctly summarized this history [8]. With strong leadership and professional society commitment, the life-threatening problems of hypoxia and airway loss were systematically evaluated and solutions were found. Technologic advances such as pulse oximeters and capnographs contributed to a safer anesthesia environment, as did the use of care teams. Improved outcomes were demonstrated in a more than tenfold reduction of anesthesia deaths, from 2/10,000 to 1/200,000 to 300,000. These improved mortality outcomes led to profession-wide adoption of the care practices that produced the improved outcomes. Anesthesia as a specialty has benefited directly from this impressive patient safety improvement by having lower malpractice insurance premiums, but the patient undergoing anesthetic care has been the primary beneficiary.

Surgery care processes

There are fundamental differences between anesthesia and surgery, insofar as anesthesia is a single discipline involving the delivery of drugs to allow surgical procedures to be done. Many of the common and life-threatening complications of anesthesia care can be simulated for trainees, and technology provides for effective monitoring to improve patient safety. On the other hand, the surgical care processes encompass preoperative evaluation and diagnosis, treatment planning, treatment execution (usually an operation), and postoperative care and follow-up. In addition to this longitudinal difference, surgery is highly specialized, and many different procedures are done within each specialty. The optimal safe system for surgical patients would address all of these areas (Fig. 1) [9].

Patient evaluation

Patients arrive on our surgical doorstep with varying degrees of evaluation already having been done. For some, the surgeon is the diagnostician. Errors at this point in the overall care process can involve poor choices in diagnostic testing or data interpretation. Cognitive error studies suggest that there are "cognitive dispositions to respond" (ie, how we respond in certain situations), and how this can lead to diagnostic error [10]. Emotional

Patient factors	Provider factors	Preoperative processes of care
Race/ethnicity	Surgeon volume	Apropriate beta blockade
Insurance coverage →	Surgeon training →	VTE prophylaxis
Socioeconomic status	(specialty training)	Preoperative antibiotic use
Co-morbidity		Preop evaluation

↓

Fewer complications	Postoperative outcomes	Intraoperative outcomes
Better outcomes	Cardiac, pulmonary	Estimated blood loss
Higher quality ←	and other complications ←	Intraoperative complications
	Failure to "rescue"	
	ICU (Intensivist-led models	
	of ICU care)	

Fig. 1. Surgical care processes. (*From* Rogers SO. The holy grail of surgical quality improvement: process measures or risk adjusted outcome? Am Surg 2006;72:1047; with permission.)

thinking or one's general attitude can lead to diagnostic error. Early diagnostic errors are common, such as locking into a diagnosis based on early information and failing to think thereafter. Probability errors are common. By "playing the odds," an unusual diagnosis can be missed. Psychiatric diagnoses may contribute to missed comorbidity, or medical problems can be incorrectly attributed to psychiatric problems.

Evidence-based medicine translated into evaluation and treatment algorithms has exploded in recent years [11]. A critical role of surgical specialty societies is to generate guidelines for general use. The Internet has facilitated dissemination of this type of information. The "practice parameters" found on the American Society of Colon and Rectal Surgeons' Web site is a good example [12].

The opposite scenario is the fully-worked-up patient who requires only a treatment plan. The decisions revolve around a knowledge of the pros and cons of whatever options exist for the condition, as related to the host-specific risk factors. Patient preference obviously comes into play as well. The ability to provide our patients in real time with probabilities of mortality and morbidity is currently fairly crude for general surgery. The National Surgical Quality Improvement Project (NSQIP) in its current form cannot yet help the patient and surgeon in the preoperative discussion of surgical risks. Aust and colleagues [13] have demonstrated the value of a mini-NSQIP type calculation that provides a more accurate preoperative mortality prediction. Improvement in risk assessment and stratification in the preoperative setting is certain to evolve, and will help surgeons make better decisions with patients who are much better informed. NSQIP data clearly demonstrate that the medical comorbidity of the patient is the biggest determinant of the cost of care for that patient [14].

The operation

Errors on the surgery service account for the slight majority of serious errors in a hospital [15]. Gawande and coworkers [16] have evaluated error on surgical services, and have shown that the operating room is the site of most errors. Wrong-site surgery is perhaps the highest-profile error. The surgical time-out, during which the patient is identified and the operation and laterality are confirmed, is a useful but imperfect scheme to limit this error [17]. Expanding this time-out to include checks for the appropriate administration of antibiotics, availability of blood and special devices or instruments, continuation of beta blockers, and venous thromboembolism (VTE) prophylaxis have proven to minimally extend the duration of the time-out, and to be remarkably effective in insuring successful completion of the important Surgical Care Improvement Project (SCIP) identified surgical care processes to actually decrease surgical site infection, myocardial infarction, and VTE [18].

Crew resource management (CRM) has its origin in aviation, and arose as a formalized effort to change the communication style in aircrafts, such that the pilot becomes an approachable part of a team, teamwork among crew members is fostered, and individual crew members are empowered [3]. The hierarchical structure, with the pilot as the sole and unquestioned decision-maker, clearly contributed to aviation disasters, and was the impetus for this change. The analogy of the aircraft to the operating room and the pilot to the surgeon is fairly obvious. CRM has been applied to the operating room, with preoperative briefings of all members of the operating team, a more open and team-oriented operating room environment, and open communication of the surgeon with the team when departures from the agreed-upon plan occur [3]. Aviation has provided other safety suggestions as well (Box 1).

There are differences in the types of error made by experienced and more junior surgeons [16]. The less experienced surgeon can be challenged by the novelty and complexity of the situation, which may lead to poor decisions and technical errors. The senior surgeon is more likely to be prone to complacency arising from years of success in performing operations in a routine fashion. The nearly automatic performance of an operation can lead to a failure to recognize the need to change something in unique circumstances. This points to the importance of appropriate mentoring and oversight of younger surgeons, and the need for vigilance and open dialogue among operating team members for all surgeons.

Box 1. Suggestions from aviation

- Require completion of CRM for hospital credentialing.
- Brief the team before an operation.
- Write standards for your organization.
- Recognize fatigue and age as factors in surgeon performance.
- Credentialing for hospital privileges should include surgical "check-rides."
- Replace morbidity and mortality (M & M) conference with mandatory reporting system to find root causes of error.
- Random drug testing for all staff

From McGreevy J, Otten T, Poggi M, et al. The challenge of changing roles and improving surgical care now: crew resource management approach. Am Surg 2006;72:1084; with permission.

Postoperative care

Standardization of care with order sets and clinical pathways is useful to prevent a forgotten order and to foster a reproducible expectation for the residents, nurses, and other care team members [19]. Acceptance by affected surgeons requires development of the orders and pathways in a collaborative fashion to be successful [3]. It is probably easier to standardize in a small community hospital or a large teaching hospital with a closed medical staff. Hospitals characterized by multiple competing practice groups that practice at multiple hospitals can pose challenges in achieving standardization. Individual practitioner or group order sets are an option, but are probably less effective overall, because nurses and other health care workers are exposed to multiple care paths and order sets with somewhat different emphases and biases. Broadly accepted order sets are, however, very valuable. An additional safety advantage of preprinted order sets is that they are always legible.

Medication error has received much attention because of the frequency, consequences, and potential preventability of those errors. In the Harvard Medical Practice Study, medication-related adverse events were the most common type of adverse event, and accounted for nearly 20% of all medical adverse events [5]. Medication errors can occur at any point along the chain of processes of ordering, transcribing, dispensing, and administering a drug. Estimates of the frequency of medication error have been variously stated as 5%, with 1% of these producing patient injury to 6.5% of adult hospital admissions [20,21]. Adverse drug events are more common on the medical services than the surgical services. At the University of Louisville Hospital, 41 medical errors were reported, covering 2187 admissions and 9828 patient days over 9 months on a surgical ward, for a frequency of 4/1000 patient days. Definite patient harm occurred in only one patient (Michael H. McCafferty, MD, unpublished data, 2005).

Among the strategies to combat medication error, computerized physician order entry (CPOE) has been proposed as a solution to minimize transcription error and to facilitate appropriate ordering, if combined with appropriate clinical support [22]. Decreased medication error has been demonstrated with CPOE, and the economic argument favoring the purchase of a CPOE system largely revolves around the savings from fewer adverse drug events [4]. There are problems with CPOE beyond the expense [23,24]. Electronic order entry is generally slower than handwritten order entry. Studies that minimize this issue are typically from the medical service with a relatively small patient census [23,25]. Introducing CPOE to a high-volume, high-acuity environment such as a busy surgical trauma service poses real challenges to residents' time usage and education, particularly with the 80-hour work week. CPOE introduces new errors, which must be confronted. As an example that the authors have witnessed, orders can be lost in cyberspace unless mechanisms to assure order takeoff exist.

Continuity of care in the teaching hospital setting has deteriorated with the 80-hour work week, making the patient handoff of major importance [26]. There are data to suggest that the benefits of a better-rested surgical resident may be more than offset by the mistakes made by covering residents who are not familiar with patients under their care [27]. The challenge, therefore, is to create an improved handoff of information to the covering residents. The solutions are local, and must take into account the information systems already in place. In highly technically advanced environments, computerized signouts that provide the necessary information for the on-call residents to function efficiently have been created [28]. In less advanced environments, manual signout with adequate time to convey appropriate information is required.

Trauma care

The trauma service is an allegedly high-risk environment from a patient safety perspective, because of the complex interactions in the field and in the hospital among various health care providers, coupled with the urgency of the need to accurately diagnose and treat the patient. The acuity of care is often very high, which creates an unusually large number of possibilities for error and patient harm. The development of the Advanced Trauma Life Support Program and the commitment of trauma surgeons and the American College of Surgeons to the problem has produced our system of trauma centers and standardization. [29]. At the local level, institutions involved in trauma care must evaluate and optimize the system from the prehospital field management through all phases of hospital care [30]. A downturn of interest in a career in trauma surgery adds a new dimension to the challenge of creating a safe environment for the care of trauma patients [31]. Through an active quality improvement program, which focuses on potentially preventable deaths and morbidity and system improvement, coupled with adherence to national society-driven better practices, trauma programs are really models for the rest of us in surgery to improve care and safety through a systems approach [30].

Strategies to improve patient safety

Morbidity and mortality conference

The M & M conference has long been the backbone of surgical teaching of residents and students. The traditional approach was to review a complication or death, to ascribe an action or actions as causative, and frequently to assign blame to one or more individuals. The study of medical error does not exonerate the individual for faulty decision-making or execution of procedures, but does recognize that most serious errors result from multiple errors within a complex system (ie, poorly designed care processes that allow for mistakes to occur) (Fig. 2) [32,33].

In this light, the educational milieu should reflect our improved understanding of error and safety. Four years ago, at the University of Louisville, we renamed and re-engineered our weekly surgical M & M conference. It is now called the Quality Improvement Conference. The resident responsible for presenting the cases reviews the potential cases with a faculty member, and the best teaching cases are selected. This eliminates the waste of

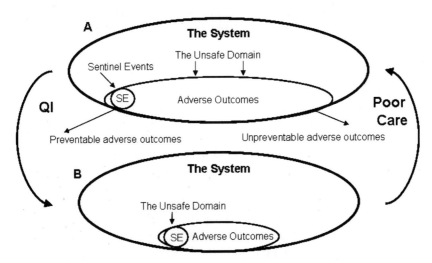

Fig. 2. Medical error processes. (*From* Khuri SF. Safety, quality and the National Surgical Quality Improvement Program. Am Surg 2006;72:997; with permission.)

valuable teaching time on cases such as nonsurvivable closed-head injury. In addition, the focus is upon improvement of patient care. Evidence-based data are presented to reinforce key teaching points. Residents are urged to evaluate cases for near misses that are used to highlight and improve patient safety. Once a month, a cost analysis case is included, wherein hospital and physician charges for a chosen case are presented to raise the awareness of students, residents, and faculty about the cost of medical care, and to stimulate improvement in efficiency and economy in health care provision [34].

Simulation

Medical simulation has tremendous appeal as a tool to educate and train people to perform procedures, and to recognize and react to threatening situations without harm to patients [35]. For example, simulation training of novices has been studied to train residents to perform colonoscopy [36,37]. The learning curve for this procedure is in excess of 100 cases. Formalized simulation training using expensive simulators can place a novice at the level of having done 30 supervised colonoscopies in patients before actually touching a patient. The Surgical Council on Resident Education has an interest in simulations as an adjunct to traditional surgical education [38].

Simulations need not be high tech and expensive. Boxes for effective laparoscopic novice skills training can be constructed inexpensively [35]. Simulation also holds promise as a tool to assess and document surgical skill. Regardless of the simulation design, there will be a continued and escalating need for simulation training for novices and experienced surgeons to meet the requirements of effective training and retraining with minimal patient risk in an environment of rapid technical advances. The latter poses real challenges to the busy practicing surgeon who needs to acquire new skills.

Outside influences

Patient safety and quality care are of concern to all health care shareholders, including employees, insurers, and consumers. The perfect storm of continually rising health care costs, the recognition of unexplained regional variations in health care, and the highly publicized 1999 publication of *To Err is Human* [6] have produced myriad efforts to improve patient safety and quality of care and to reduce health care costs. The Leapfrog Group was formed in 2000 by large employers to attempt to leverage purchasing power as a change agent in health care [39]. Representing more than 170 entities that purchase health care for over 37 million people, this organization has clout. It has established some quality practices for hospitals, which include CPOE to decrease medication error, critical care physician oversight of intensive care unit patients, and evidence-based (volume-related) hospital referral [40]. Hospitals want to comply with these "quality practices" despite remaining issues of cost, complexity, and unintended consequences of CPOE, the logistical difficulties of intensivist preeminence in the intensive care unit (ICU), and questions about the validity of the surgical volume and quality relationship [41].

The National Quality Forum (NQF) is a private, not-for-profit membership organization created to develop and implement a national strategy for health care quality measurements and reporting [42,43]. The NQF was founded in 1999 in response to a 1998 report entitled *President's Advisory Commission on Consumer Protection and Quality in the Health Care Industry*. The NQF member organizations represent consumers, health professionals (eg, American College of Surgeons), providers, insurers, purchasers, and research and quality improvement groups. The NQF has established 22 national priorities for health care quality measurement and reporting, 2 of which are patient safety and cancer [42]. The NQF accepted a recommendation by the American College of Surgeons that the removal of at least 12 lymph nodes with operations for colorectal cancer is a legitimate quality indicator [44]. As an isolated quality measure, this is certainly not meaningful in the absence of other outcomes measures (eg, mortality and anastomotic leak rates). It is, however, a simple measure of the sort that insurers like because it is inexpensively obtained. Interestingly, United Healthcare has invited surgeons in the authors' area to voluntarily submit five deidentified cases documenting that this single "quality" standard has been met. Oncology nurses working for that company will "be contacting United Healthcare members who have a new diagnosis of colorectal carcinoma to educate them about the importance of lymph node sampling. During this discussion they will provide names of all participating surgeons who have demonstrated, through their application responses, their experience in removing 12 or more nodes in at least 5 operations for colorectal cancer." (Letter from Allen E. Grimes, MD, United Healthcare, 2006). In addition to being void of meaning as an isolated quality measure, this does not necessarily reflect surgical technical competence in performing the resection, because the effort of the pathologist has a more direct bearing on the number of lymph nodes identified for analysis. Preoperative chemotherapy and radiation for rectal cancer is commonplace, and the lymph node yield by even the best pathologists is very much lower [45].

Centers for Medicaid and Medicare Services (CMS) identified surgical site infection (SSI), VTE, and perioperative myocardial infarction as three sources of postoperative M & M that could be substantially improved by the application of evidence-based interventions. This resulted in the SCIP [46]. Kentucky surgeons participated in the SCIP pilot, which was designed to measure processes related to these outcomes (ie, appropriate antibiotic use: choice, timing, duration), VTE prophylaxis, and β-blockade. This approach to quality improvement in surgical care emphasizes process improvement and local system redesign as needed to achieve improved compliance with these proven care elements. The results of that pilot trial have been published. The American Medical Association has agreed with congressional leaders to establish quality measures [47]. If this plan is passed, CMS will seek quality measures for many specialties.

There are other significant organizations that are committed to improving patient safety and quality, but the point is that there are strong forces of change that are being driven by health care purchasers (commercial and governmental) and consumers. Expectations grow for increasing accountability and transparency from health care providers [26]. The Agency for Healthcare Research and Quality (AHRQ) has an extensive Web site, part of which is oriented to consumers [48]. Questions to ask your surgeon are among the sections. It is clear that consumers are now armed with advice and data, and that they continually seek even more objective data [46].

Challenges and solutions

Patient safety and improving the quality of care are rightfully subjects that the health care system, with strong physician leadership, must address. Our collective failure to do so will be met with solutions being thrust upon us from outside entities that have a legitimate and serious interest in containing costs, reducing variations in care, and developing and demanding quality in health care. In a nonuniform health care system, as exists in the United States, solutions are complex, and require involvement at the national, regional, and local levels.

Quality in health care relates to achieving favorable outcomes in a cost-effective and patient-centered fashion. Process measures are frequently used as surrogate markers of quality because processes determine outcomes, and process measures are more numerous and easily determined [46]. Some of the difficulties in quality measurement in surgery include the wide range of surgical procedures for which measures are needed, choosing a core of meaningful measures, keeping data acquisitions simple, minimizing data acquisition costs, deciding who will pay for data acquisition, incorporating meaningful patient risk stratification, and understanding the use of the data. Potential uses of individual surgeon quality data include quality improvement initiatives, pay-for-performance (P4P), maintenance of certification (MOC), and consumer evaluation [46,49,50].

The NSQIP is a Veterans Administration (VA)-validated, risk-adjusted outcomes database that now includes over 1 million surgical procedures [51]. It has now been validated outside of the VA system. It includes the gathering of 95 pieces of data from the preoperative, intraoperative, and postoperative periods. Specially trained nurses gather the data, which are forwarded to a data analysis center. Outcomes are calculated as observed:expected (O/E) ratios for M & M. The M & M for surgical procedures in the VA system has improved dramatically since the NSQIP was begun (Figs. 3, 4) [52].

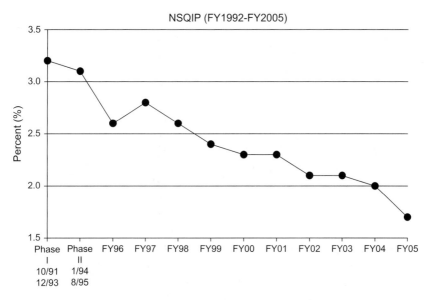

Fig. 3. Trends in unadjusted 30-day mortality rate for major noncardiac surgery (all operations). (*From* DePalma RG. Surgical quality programs in the Veterans Health Administration. Am Surg 2006;72:1002; with permission.)

Although this project demonstrates the power of data and their favorable effect on surgical outcomes, NSQIP is expensive and labor intensive. A simpler risk stratification methodology that has more upfront (preoperative) utility and less expense is desirable, unless NSQIP per se becomes a governmental mandate.

Surgical specialties and their national societies must determine and endorse a risk stratification scheme that is applicable to major surgical procedures. The virtue of the six-variable scheme described by Aust and colleagues [13] is its simplicity and correlation with NSQIP predictions of mortality. Specialties should also determine appropriate process and outcomes measures for major surgical procedures. Reasonable process measures include the SCIP measure to decrease SSI, VTE, and perioperative myocardial infarction. Important outcomes measures are procedure-specific and should be chosen by surgeons.

As mentioned previously, the development and dissemination of evidence-based practices is an important role of specialty societies. Quality indicators for less complex procedures such as colonoscopy differ. Using the colonoscopy example, it would probably suffice to focus on appropriate indications, cecal and terminal ileum intubation rates proven by photo documentation, and incidence of complications requiring hospitalization. The latter would capture perforations, significant bleeding, and significant sedation-related complications.

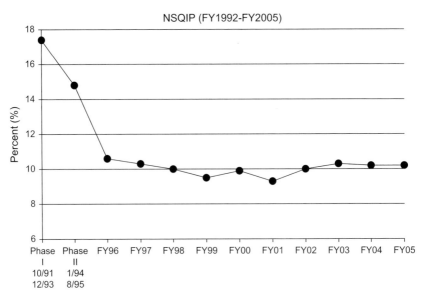

Fig. 4. Trends in unadjusted 30-day morbidity rate for major noncardiac surgery (all operations). Actual mortality and morbidity trends for the National Surgery Quality Improvement
Program (15 years from inception through fiscal year 2005). (*From* DePalma RG. Surgical
quality programs in the Veterans Health Administration. Am Surg 2006;72:1002; with
permission.)

Leadership is also important at the local and regional levels. There is no
simple formula to this, but it requires physician commitment. Quality Surgical
Solutions (QSS) was formed in 1997 in Kentucky by a group of surgical
specialists who foresaw the importance of surgeon leadership in defining quality care and better practices [46]. This group was unique insofar as it involved
surgical specialists from urban and rural practices, all of whom shared a common vision of improving care for their patients. QSS has addressed quality and
economic issues such as the decreasing cost of laparoscopic cholecystectomy
with reusable instruments, decreasing the use of cardiology consultation in
conjunction with anesthesia evaluation and agreement, and decreasing the
use of expensive antiemetics [53,54]. QSS has a database of a wide variety of
surgical procedures, which made QSS appealing to CMS when the SCIP pilot
was contemplated. QSS, in conjunction with Health Care Excel (the regional
quality improvement organization) accrued and analyzed in excess of 5000
cases for SCIP. QSS currently has a grant to help much smaller hospitals
implement SCIP care processes. This decade-long track record of involvement
in surgical-quality–related issues has helped the participating surgeons and
their hospitals benefit from the collective wisdom of the group, and to lead
instead of being led.

At the individual hospital level, there are numerous opportunities to
improve patient safety. As was mentioned, the expanded surgical time-out

incorporates the confirmation of important care processes into an already-established pause to identify the patient and procedure. Real-time monitoring of this is helpful to establish a pattern of compliance, and to provide feedback to the operating room personnel. The authors' group has established a monthly quality and safety meeting with middle management at University of Louisville Hospital over the past 18 months. This has been a very useful forum to discuss safety issues, prioritize actionable programs, and to report progress in our hospital.

Education of residents and students via the retooled M & M conference has helped to inculcate the next generation of surgeons with the jargon, thought processes, and importance of safety and quality. Including all health care workers in the process using a positive deviance model has been remarkably effective in decreasing methicillin-resistant *Staphylococcus aureus* (MRSA) transmission at the Pittsburgh Veterans Administration Hospital, and is being instituted at the University of Louisville Hospital [55]. The forums of surgical grand rounds and the local surgical societies have been used to further education at a local level.

Summary

Patient safety and quality of care are inextricably linked. Surgery encompasses such a wide spectrum of diagnosis, treatment, postoperative care, and outpatient follow-up of so many illnesses that quality improvement and patient safety opportunities are numerous and potentially overwhelming. The study of error can be applied across all components of the care process, and offers many points of study to improve patient safety. Possible roles of individual surgeon leaders, local organizations, and national organizations in the arena of patient safety and quality improvement have been described. The current emphasis on patient safety and quality improvement is also linked to the economics of medical care [56,57]. A fundamental premise is that appropriate and safely delivered health care is less expensive. In our current climate, this emphasis on quality and safety will remain a high priority. Surgeon leadership at all levels is key to our professional viability.

References

[1] Millenson ML. Trust me, I'm a doctor. In: Demanding medical excellence. Chicago: University of Chicago Press; 1985. p. 141–7.

[2] Russell TR, Jones RS. American College of Surgeons remains committed to patient safety. Am Surg 2006;72:1005–9.

[3] McGreevy J, Otten T, Poggi M, et al. The challenge of changing roles and improving surgical care now: crew resource management approach. Am Surg 2006;72:1082–7.

[4] Rhodes RS. Invited commentary: analyzing adverse medical events—It's the system!. Surgery 2003;133(6):624–6.

[5] Leape LL, Brennan TA, Laird N, et al. The nature of adverse events in hospitalized patients: results of the Harvard Medical Practice Study II. N Engl J Med 1991;324:377–84.

[6] Kohn LT, Corrigan JM, Donaldson MS, editors. To err is human. Washington, DC: National Academy Press; 1999.

[7] Wennberg JE, Cooper MM, editors. The Dartmouth atlas of health care in the United States. Chicago, IL: American Hospital Publishing, Inc.; 1996.

[8] Lanier W. A three decade perspective on anesthesia safety. Am Surg 2006;72:985–9.

[9] Rogers SO. The holy grail of surgical quality improvement: process measures or risk adjusted outcome? Am Surg 2006;72:1046–50.

[10] Croskerry P. The importance of cognitive errors in diagnosis and strategies to minimize them. Acad Med 2003;78(8):775–82.

[11] Maier RV. What the surgeon of tomorrow needs to know about evidence-based surgery. Arch Surg 2006;141:317–23.

[12] American Society of Colon and Rectal Surgeons. Available at: http://www.fascrs.org/displaycommon.cfm?an=18subarticlenbr=63. Accessed May 19, 2007.

[13] Aust JB, Henderson W, Khuri S, et al. The impact of operative complexity on patient risk factors. Ann Surg 2005;241(6):1024–8.

[14] Davenport DL, Henderson WG, Khuri ST, et al. Preoperative risk factors and surgical complexity are more predictive of costs than postoperative complications: a case study using the National Surgical Quality Improvement Program (NSQIP) database. Ann Surg 2005;242(4):463–8.

[15] Gawande AA, Thomas EJ, Zinner MJ. The incidence and nature of surgical adverse events in Colorado and Utah in 1992. Surgery 1999;126:66–75.

[16] Gawande AA, Zinner MJ, Studdert DM. Analysis of errors reported by surgeons at three teaching hospitals. Surgery 2003;133(6):614–21.

[17] Crokcan RJ. Wrong site surgery. In: Manuel BM, Nova PF, editors. Surgical patient safety: essential information for surgeons in today's environment. Chicago: The American College of Surgeons; 2004. p. 107–17.

[18] Altpeter T, Luckhardt K, Lewis JN, et al. Expanded surgical time out: a key to real-time data collection and quality improvement. J American College of Surgeons 2007;204(4):527–32.

[19] Polk HC. The evolution of guidelines toward standards of practice. Am Surg 2006;72:1017–20.

[20] Bates DW, Boyle DC, VanderVliet MB, et al. Relationship between medication errors and adverse drug events. J Gen Intern Med 1995;10:199–205.

[21] Bates DW, Cullen D, Laird N, et al. Incidence of adverse drug events and potential adverse drug events: implications for prevention. JAMA 1995;274:29–34.

[22] Bates DW, Leape LL, Cullen DJ, et al. Effect of computerized physician order entry and a team intervention on prevention of serious medication errors. JAMA 1998;280:1311–6.

[23] Han YY, Carcillo JA, Shekhar TV, et al. Unexpected increased mortality after implementation of a commercially sold computerized physician order entry system. Pediatrics 2005;116(6):1506–12.

[24] Nebeker JR, Hoffman JM, Weir CR, et al. High rates of adverse drug events in a highly computerized hospital. Archives of Internal Medicine 2005;165(10):1111–6.

[25] Tierney WM, Miller ME, Overhage JM, et al. Physician inpatient order writing on microcomputer workstations. JAMA 1993;269(3):379–83.

[26] Polk HC Jr. Presidential address: quality, safety and transparency. Ann Surg 2005;242(3):293–301.

[27] Petersen LA, Brennan TA, Cook EE, et al. Does housestaff discontinuity of care increase the risk for preventable adverse events? Ann Intern Med 1994;121:866–72.

[28] Van Eaton EG, Horrath KD, Loser WB, et al. A randomized, controlled trial evaluating the impact of a computerized rounding and sign-out system on continuity of care and resident work hours. J Am Coll Surg 2005;200:538–45.

[29] Course overview: the purpose, history and concept of the ATLS program for doctors. In: ATLS Advanced Trauma Life Support. Chicago: The American College of Surgeons; 2004.

[30] Mackenzie RC, Rhodes M. Patient safety in trauma care. In: Manuel BM, Nova PF, editors. Surgical patient safety. Chicago: The American College of Surgeons; 2004. p. 61–77.

[31] Richardson JD, Miller F. Will future surgeons be interested in trauma care? Results of a resident survey. J Trauma 1992;32:229–35.

[32] Spencer FC. Human error in hospitals and industrial accidents: current concepts. J Am Coll Surg 2000;191(4):410–8.

[33] Khuri SF. Safety, quality and the National Surgical Quality Improvement Program. Am Surg 2006;72:994–6.

[34] McCafferty MH, Polk HC Jr. Addition of "near-miss" cases enhances a quality improvement conference. Arch Surg 2004;139:216–7.

[35] Dunkin B, Adrolls GL, Apelgren K, et al. Surgical simulation: a current review. Surg Endosc 2007;21:357–66.

[36] Cass OW, Freeman ML, Peine CJ, et al. Objective evaluation of endoscopy skills during training. Ann Intern Med 1993;118(1):40–4.

[37] Marshall JB. Technical proficiency of trainees performing colonoscopy: a learning curve. Gastrointest Endosc 1995;42(4):287–91.

[38] Bell RH. Surgical council on resident education: a new organization devoted to graduate surgical education. J Am Coll Surg 2007;204(3):341–6.

[39] The Leap Frog Group. Available at: http://leapfroggroup.org. Accessed March 12, 2006.

[40] Leapfrog Hospital Quality and Safety Survey. Available at: http://www.leapfroggroup. org/for_hospitals/leapfrog_hospital_quality_and_safety_survey_copy/leapfrog_safety_ prectices. Accessed July 10, 2006.

[41] Christian CK, Gutofson ML, Betensky RA, et al. The Leapfrog volume criteria may fall short in identifying high-quality surgical centers. Ann Surg 2003;238(4):447–57.

[42] Available at: http://www.qualityforum.org/about/home.html. Accessed March 12, 2006.

[43] National Quality Forum (NQF). National priorities for healthcare quality measurement and reporting. Washington, DC: NQF; 2004.

[44] Available at: http://www.fascrs.org/associations/1843/files/ASCRSNewsSpring06.pdf. Accessed May 8, 2006.

[45] Sermier A, Gervaz P, Egger JF, et al. Lymph node retrieval in abdominoperineal surgical specimens is radiation time-dependent. World J Surg Oncol 2006;4:29–32.

[46] Polk HC, Lewis JN, Garrison RN, et al. Process and outcome measures in specialty surgery: early steps in defining quality. Bull Am Coll Surg 2005;90(2):9–15.

[47] Lubell J. AMA performance pact imposes hard deadline. Surgery News 2006;4:1,3.

[48] Available at: http://www.ahcpr.gov/qual/. Accessed March 12, 2006.

[49] Friesen J. Paying for quality: making policy and practice work for patients. Bull Am Coll Surg 2005;90(11):8–13.

[50] Russell TR. From my perspective. Bull Am Coll Surg 2000;90(5):4–6.

[51] Khuri SF, Daley J, Henderson W, et al. The Department of Veterans Affairs' NSQIP: The first national, validated, outcome-based, risk adjusted, and peer-controlled program for measurement and enhancement for the quality of surgical care. Ann Surg 1998;228:491–507.

[52] DePalma RG. Surgical quality programs in the Veterans Health Administration. Am Surg 2006;72:999–1004.

[53] Allen JW, Polk HC. A study of added costs of laparoscopic cholecystectomy based on surgery preference cards. Am Surg 2002;68(5):474–6.

[54] Shively EH, Heine RJ, Schell RH, et al. Practicing surgeons lead in quality care, safety, and cost control. Ann Surg 2004;239(6):752–62.

[55] Buscell P. Plexus versus the bacteria. Emerging: the MRSA issues 2006;(winter):9–18.

[56] Hall RL, Campbell DA, Phillips LR, et al. Evaluating individual surgeons based on total hospital cases: evidence for variation in both total costs and volatility of costs. J Am College of Surgeons 2006;202(4):565–76.

[57] Dimick JB, Weeks WB, Karia RJ, et al. Who pays for poor surgical quality? Building a business case for quality improvement. J Am Coll Surg 2006;202(6):933–7.

ELSEVIER
SAUNDERS

Surg Clin N Am 87 (2007) 883–887

SURGICAL
CLINICS OF
NORTH AMERICA

Employers Flex Their Muscles as Health Care Purchasers

Suzanne Delbanco, PhD

The Leapfrog Group, 1801 K Street NW, Suite 701-L, Washington, DC 20006, USA

On one hand, the health care market place is unlike any other. It deals not with widgets, but with lives. On the other hand, the health care marketplace is just like others: its proper functioning depends on basic market forces and signals. Patients and other purchasers of health care, like large employers, need to exert those forces and send strong signals about their needs.

But up until now, it seems as if the patient, who stands the most to gain or lose, has largely been a quiet recipient of whatever care comes his or her way. Employers and other organizations and agencies who purchase health care on behalf of patients also have significantly underutilized their leverage in the system. If there is any hope of improving the value of care by raising quality and shaving the upward trend of health care costs, the health care system needs both to play a more active role.

Engaged health care purchasers—both individual and group—can stimulate some good, healthy competition in the health care system, and competition needs to be based on results. To determine results, we need accepted measures of quality and efficiency that make sense. Then, performance on those measures must be disclosed publicly. Only when this information is available to consumers and other purchasers of health care will they be able to make informed choices and reward effective and efficient health care providers.

Banding together for greater market force

Like individuals, employers are consumers and purchasers, but on a much larger scale. Many of the nation's largest employers and other purchasers of health care are members of The Leapfrog Group, a coalition working to improve the delivery and overall value of health care. In 2000, The Leapfrog Group was formed, and its members agreed on four premises about the ailing health care system:

E-mail address: ksong@leapfroggroup.org

doi:10.1016/j.suc.2007.07.011   *surgical.theclinics.com*

- American health care remains far below obtainable levels of basic safety, quality, and overall customer value.
- The health industry will improve more rapidly if purchasers better recognize and reward superior safety and overall value (via provider ratings and incentive and reward initiatives).
- Adherence to certain purchasing principles by a critical mass of America's largest employers will jump-start improvements in health care.
- These principles should not only seek superior overall value from providers, but also focus on a few specific innovations that offer high-impact and immediate "leaps" forward in quality and safety.

On behalf of the tens of millions of Americans for whom its members buy health benefits, Leapfrog aims to use its leverage for two main purposes. First, to convince the health care system to share standard measurements of performance fully and openly with both health professionals and the public. This helps create an environment that is far more conducive to re-engineering how health care is delivered. Second, to promote high-value health care through the use of financial rewards, such as pay-for-performance (P4P). Augmenting this, Leapfrog helps its members employ another tactic to affect market forces—implementing financial incentives that encourage employees to choose high-performing health care providers over ones that offer poorer quality and efficiency.

Using the vehicle of hospital quality and safety, Leapfrog hopes to be a catalyst for integrating these changes into the permanent fabric of the health care system, and to drive improvements in care at the same time.

Pushing for better care

Based on strong evidence that they can make a vital difference to patients, Leapfrog promotes specific practices, or "leaps," in US hospitals. When Leapfrog began its work, employers sought advice from leading quality improvement experts in the search for the equivalents of antilock brakes, seat belts, and airbags for hospital care. Independent scientific evidence points to several practices that could both improve outcomes significantly and be easily understood by the average patient when choosing among hospitals. Through the ongoing, voluntary Leapfrog Hospital Quality and Safety Survey, we track hospitals implementation of the following practices:

- Computerized physician order entry (CPOE). With a CPOE system in place, physicians enter patient prescriptions and other orders into computers linked to error-prevention software. CPOE can save $9 to $16 per patient per hospital day. Implementing CPOE in all US hospitals would save about $1.5 billion annually.
- Intensive care unit (ICU) physician staffing. Patient care in the ICU is managed by doctors with special training in ICU care, known as

intensivists. Direct savings and indirect productivity benefits from ICU physician staffing in all US hospitals with ICUs would be approximately $3.4 billion annually. On a per-hospital basis, the average net savings attributable to ICU physician staffing is about $578 per ICU bed-day (for a midsize, 12-bed ICU unit), and length-of-stay is reduced by 1 to 2 days.

- Evidence-based hospital referral. Leapfrog's Hospital Quality and Safety Survey asks hospitals how well they perform seven high-risk procedures and care for two high-risk neonatal conditions. This information is meant to guide patients to hospitals with a proven track record. For instance, the survey asks how many times a year a hospital and its surgeons perform each of the procedures; it also asks those with neonatal ICUs how many infants they typically care for each day. For some of the procedures and conditions, hospitals can report their adherence to patient care processes that are correlated with high quality, as well as risk-adjusted outcomes data.
- Leapfrog Safe Practices Score. Leapfrog scores hospitals' progress on 27 National Quality Forum (NQF) safe practices (with the first 3 practices above, these complete the full set of 30 NQF-endorsed safe practices). These practices include the prevention of surgical site infections and implementing the Universal Protocol for Preventing Wrong Site, Wrong Procedure, Wrong Person Surgery for all invasive procedures.

These practices are a practical first step in using purchasing power to improve health quality and safety. There is overwhelming scientific evidence that implementation of these safety and quality practices will significantly reduce preventable medical mistakes. Although implementing them may be challenging, many hospitals have already proven that it is feasible and effective. Furthermore, employing just the first three practices in all US hospitals can save our health care system up to $41.5 billion per year.

Leapfrog posts survey responses publicly on our Web site at www.leapfroggroup.org, and disseminates them further to consumers through our members, major health plans, and the media. Health plans, purchasers, and consumers can use Survey results to help select among hospitals.

The Survey was revolutionary when we launched it, creating unprecedented access to hospital-specific information for consumers. Today, it enjoys more company. As a catalyst, the Survey sparked other initiatives to create greater transparency in health care by collecting further information both from hospitals and physicians at both the state and national levels, including those led by the public sector.

Paying for better care

Leapfrog does not stop at figuring out how well providers deliver care. Better providers deserve better pay and more business. And, of course, health care doesn't happen only in hospitals. It is provided in numerous other venues, particularly physician offices.

Two years ago, Leapfrog launched the Leapfrog Hospital Rewards Program to create ways for employers and health plans to provide rewards to hospitals that demonstrate both high quality of care and efficient use of resources, and incentives to patients to seek care from these high-performing providers. Health plans and employers that implement the program are able to determine which providers should receive bonus financial payments or enjoy increased market share by having patients directed to their doors. The program initially focuses on five clinical areas that represent a significant proportion of hospital admissions and expenditures among the commercially-insured population: (1) coronary artery bypass graft (CABG), (2) percutaneous coronary intervention, (3) acute myocardial infarction (AMI), (4) community acquired pneumonia (CAP), and (5) deliveries/newborn care. Together, these five clinical areas account for 20% of commercial spending on inpatient services and 33% of commercial admissions to hospitals. The quality measures used for each of these conditions are endorsed by the NQF.

The measure of resource use, developed by Thomson Healthcare, has a completely transparent methodology and looks at severity-adjusted length of stay and readmission rates for each of the clinical areas. Actual cost or payment information would bolster the efficiency measures, and each implementer of the program can incorporate these data on its own.

Actuarial work done by Towers Perrin demonstrates that not only do these five clinical areas represent a significant proportion of commercial inpatient spending, but they also represent significant opportunity for quality and efficiency improvement. Analyses of national quality and efficiency data for CABG, AMI, and CAP show that, across these three clinical areas, only 5% to 8% of hospitals fall into the program's top performance group. These top performers also have average payments 25% to 35% lower than the national average payment for each respective clinical area.

Another tool we recently unveiled is the return on investment (ROI) Estimator. This tool is designed for use by employers and health plans to estimate the costs and financial benefits of implementing the Leapfrog Hospital Rewards Program. The ROI Estimator shows the potential return on investment, in terms of both lives and money saved, from implementing a P4P program that rewards hospitals for providing high-quality, high-value care in the five clinical areas noted above. The tool calculates financial and clinical returns as hospital performance improves on these measures. Freely available at www.ROIEstimator.com, the Leapfrog Group hopes that the ROI Estimator will be used as an open source tool for organizations to create their own tools to calculate the benefits and savings from other pay-for-performance programs.

Employers are looking to align financial incentives with quality, but in an era when health care costs continue to rise, it may be unpalatable to pay more, so providing rewards in the form of market share can be more appealing and financially feasible. Leapfrog member Boeing rolled out a pilot program a few years ago using Leapfrog hospital data to provide financial incentives for employees to go to "Leapfrog-compliant" hospitals. Employees in Boeing's traditional medical plan who choose hospitals that meet Leapfrog's standards have a 100% hospitalization benefit. Those choosing other hospitals receive only a 95% benefit.

In the outpatient setting, Leapfrog is working with the Agency for Healthcare Research and Quality, the Centers for Medicare and Medicaid Services, and Bridges to Excellence to ensure that proven practices and technology are used in this setting to improve the quality and efficiency of care. Physicians in particular markets are encouraged to participate in the Bridges to Excellence reward program. In this program, physician performance is assessed for adherence to practice guidelines for patients who have diabetes and cardiovascular disease, as well as for patient education and use of health information technology and other areas.

To further encourage the practice of rewarding better health care, we have also created the Leapfrog Incentives and Rewards Compendium found at http://www.leapfroggroup.org/leapfrog_compendium. This searchable database catalogs efforts across the country to use both financial and non-financial incentives and rewards to motivate quality improvement. Many of these programs target physicians. The good news is that purchasers and payers are beginning to pay more for improvements in the quality of care. But that accompanies increased scrutiny of whether care adheres to evidence-based guidelines.

By diving in headfirst as proactive health care purchasers, employers hope to bring a much-needed perspective into the discourse on and practice of improving the American health care system. The Leapfrog Group believes strongly that without collaboration among all parties—providers, insurers, consumers, government—lasting and meaningful change is impossible.

ELSEVIER
SAUNDERS

Surg Clin N Am 87 (2007) 889–901

SURGICAL
CLINICS OF
NORTH AMERICA

The Role of the Expert Witness

Laurance Jerrold, DDS, JD, ABO

*School of Orthodontics, Jacksonville University, 2800 University Boulevard North,
Jacksonville, FL 32211, USA*

The role of expert witnesses in medical malpractice litigation is often misunderstood. Much maligned, the expert has been the subject of castigation by a range of people, from his professional colleagues to the jurists who preside over his testimony. From an academic perspective, the expert witness is a necessary evil and his denigration is his own doing, for the expert is a neutral character who creates his own professional persona. This purpose of this article is to serve as a primer for those interested in understanding the role that the expert is supposed to play in litigation, and the factors surrounding his activities.

Before turning to the specifics of the expert's duties, anyone wanting to really understand the subject must first come to grips with the legal elements that a plaintiff must prove to succeed in a cause of action based on professional negligence. After that, one needs to become familiar with what the standard of care is and how it is established. Once those two concepts are clear, one can then fully appreciate the role of the expert witness.

Overview of the legal system

Before tackling the first issue, a brief overview of the trial advocacy system is in order. To put it in its most simplistic terms there are opposing parties, a judge, and a jury. The parties are adversarial, the judge is the trier of law, and the jury is the trier of fact. It is the judge who will decide all questions of law. These might be such issues as what statutes apply in a certain situation, if the suit was brought in a timely manner, what evidence is admissible, and who may testify, and to what. All of these questions may seriously affect the outcome of the case; but unless it is a bench trial, one with no jury, the judge does not decide the facts of a case, does not decide whether one did or did not commit malpractice, will not evaluate the extent of any injury suffered; and will not, except to modify grossly unconscionable

E-mail address: ljerrol@ju.edusyn

0039-6109/07/$ - see front matter © 2007 Elsevier Inc. All rights reserved.
doi:10.1016/j.suc.2007.07.010 *surgical.theclinics.com*

jury awards, determine the monetary amount awarded. All of the above noted queries are determined by the trier of fact, the jury. It is the jury who the expert witness is there to help.

What is negligence?

Returning to the elements that a plaintiff must prove to succeed in a malpractice suit, one must first look at the definition of negligence. Black's Law Dictionary [1] defines negligence as:

> Negligence is the failure to use such care as a reasonably prudent and careful person would use under similar circumstances; it is the doing of some act which a person of ordinary prudence would not have done under similar circumstances or failure to do what a person of ordinary prudence would have done under similar circumstances.
>
> ... The term refers only to that delinquency which results whenever a man fails to exhibit the care which he ought to exhibit, whether it be slight, ordinary, or great. It is characterized chiefly by inadvertence, thoughtlessness, inattention, and the like, while "wantonness" or "recklessness" is characterized by willfulness. The law of negligence is founded on reasonable conduct or reasonable care under all circumstances of [a] particular case. [The] doctrine of negligence rests on [a] duty of every person to exercise due care in his conduct toward others from which injury may result [2].

Negligence is a type of tort; a civil wrong, independent of contract, based on a special relationship or implied by law. The special relationship is the doctor–patient relationship, without which no duty is owed to anyone. The laws of tort are established in part by case law, examples of which would be cases from higher courts providing legal precedent; or by statute, defining such things as statutes of limitations, who may be qualified as an expert, and the like.

The first element is that the plaintiff must prove that the defendant was under a duty to have conformed to an accepted standard of care. The second element is that the defendant breached that duty. The third element is that actual injuries or losses were suffered by the plaintiff. The final element is that one's breach of this defined duty was the direct or proximate cause of the injuries sustained. These elements do not have to be proven beyond a reasonable doubt; the level of proof required is merely that exhibited by a preponderance of the evidence.

What is the standard of care? Where do these standards come from? Who determines exactly what the standard of care is in a given situation? Do the courts set the standards of care? No, except in extreme circumstances. Do our professional training programs determine it? There might be institutional regulations that apply, but again, for the most part, that is not where our standards of care come from. Do professional journals and texts set the standard? Unless they are considered authoritative, no, because they can be challenged. Also, over time, in certain circumstances they become outdated and therefore lack applicability. Do professional organizations determine the standard of care? To the extent that guidelines and parameters of care have been established they may play some role. Does the legislature set the standard of care? Again, in some situations laws have been established that govern certain aspects of the delivery of health care; but these are not the main wells from which the standards of professional care are drawn. Enter the role of the expert witness.

Why experts are necessary

Vermont, for example, measures the standard of care by the degree of care, skill, diligence, and knowledge commonly possessed and exercised by a reasonable, careful, and prudent professional practicing in that state [3]. As a general rule, expert testimony is required to show both the standard of care and a breach of that standard [4]. Suppose you are a layperson assigned to the jury on a medical malpractice case, and you have to decide whether or not a doctor conformed to certain standard of care, and if not, the extent of the plaintiff's injuries. How do you do this? The answer is through the use of expert testimony.

The expert witness will first interpret the medical terminology and testimony into basic English for the jury. The witness will then provide the jury with an opinion on what he believes the standard of care to be. He or she will then follow with an opinion as to whether or not the doctor's conduct conformed to that standard of care, or whether the physician breached the standard. The expert will then provide an explanation of the injury sustained in terms of severity, permanency, ramifications, and so forth. Finally, and most importantly, the expert will provide an opinion as to whether the breach of the duty was the direct or proximate cause of the plaintiff's injury. All of this is done to aid the jury in their deliberations in deciding whether or not the plaintiff has met his or her burden by proving by a preponderance of the evidence that all four of the elements stated above were met. A plaintiff's expert's testimony will correlate precisely with each of those elements, whereas the defendant's expert will endeavor to show the jury that one or more of the elements has not been met.

The District of Columbia, like many other jurisdictions, requires that if the subject in question is so distinctly related to some type of science, profession or occupation, and the knowledge and information relating to the issues at hand are beyond the ken of the average layperson, then expert testimony will be required to establish the standard of care and issues relating to causation [5].

Who can be an expert?

Before the trier of fact ever gets to hear an expert witness testify, the trier of law must qualify the expert as such. An Illinois case [6] succinctly summarizes the qualifications necessary. First the expert must be a "licensed member of the school of medicine about which he proposes to testify." After that, the expert must show that "he is familiar with the methods, procedures, and treatments ordinarily observed by other physicians, in either the defendant's community or a similar community." The trial judge now has the discretion to determine whether or not the proposed expert is competent to testify as such. The court will make the ultimate determination not on the doctor's credentials, schooling, professional accomplishments, and the like, but instead will focus on just two things: whether the alleged negligence concerns matters within the expert's knowledge and observation, and whether or not the expert is able to aid the trier of fact in reaching a conclusion on the issues. Once qualified, the opposing party has the opportunity to refute the expert's testimony by pointing out any infirmities in his opinion or by questioning the expert's competency to testify on the issues at hand. A case from Washington [7] notes that its Rules of Evidence (ER 702) follow the Federal Rules, which state

> If scientific, technical, or other specialized knowledge will assist the trier of fact to understand the evidence or to determine a fact in issue, a witness qualified as an expert by knowledge, skill, experience, training, or education, may testify thereto in the form of an opinion or otherwise.

Determining the standard of care

Geographic considerations

Now that we have the idea of what an expert does and how one becomes an expert, let us look at some very common language regarding the standard of care. North Carolina requires its health care professionals to perform their ministrations in accordance with the standards of practice among members of the same health care profession with similar training and experience, who are situated in the same or similar community as the defendant at the time the alleged negligence occurred [8]. The expert witness must be either in the same field of practice, or the expert must be so familiar with the field or practice in question that he is able to testify as to the standard of care in that particular field of medicine, and to be able to determine whether or not a breach of that standard has occurred [9].

Mississippi, on the other hand, has defined its standard of care as that level of degree of care, skill, diligence, and so forth, as practiced by reasonably careful, skillful, diligent and prudent practitioners within Mississippi *and for a reasonable distance adjacent to state boundaries* [10]. The court went on to say in the same case that an expert witness who is knowledgeable of and familiar with the statewide standard of care cannot have his testimony stricken merely because he did not practice within the state. On the other hand, an appellate court in Louisiana [11] noted that an expert must be familiar with the degree of care ordinarily exercised by physicians in, if not the same community, at least similar ones. In that case, the court noted that not only did the plaintiff's expert never practice in Louisiana, though he did practice in an adjoining state, he also did not receive his medical education in Louisiana, nor was there evidence presented that the expert attempted to demographically compare the locale of the defendant doctor to the locale in which he practiced to determine similarity of the locales. His testimony was not allowed.

When Montana modified its locality rule [12], it did so with due consideration being paid to the difficulty encountered in procuring expert witnesses in more rural areas. Bolstered by an amicus brief filed by the Montana Medical Association stating in part that altering the then existing law would increase the availability of expert witnesses, the court concluded that given the necessity to obtain the required expert testimony, the standard of care needed to be changed from a rigid locality rule to a more geographically expanded one, because the "similar communities" in Montana were too restrictive. Tennessee, on the other hand, besides adhering to a locality rule to establish the standard of care, reinforces that rationale by requiring experts testifying in its courts to come from within the state or from a contiguous state [13].

General qualifications

It should be obvious by now that every state defines the standard of care similarly, however many nuances abound. Essentially, we are dealing with three elements. The doctor will possess a requisite amount of "SKEE," an acronym for skill, knowledge, experience, and expertise. Although we may argue as to exactly what level of SKEE one needs to possess, such argument is pointless, because in the first place, one is required to have a license to practice. Secondly, that license is achieved in part by passing some type of qualifying examination, depending on the profession. And third, all examinations have a minimal passing grade. Although we may not like to think about it in these terms, for Mississippi and many other jurisdictions, SKEE is the possession of merely the minimal amount of competency regarding the qualities denoted [14]. The next element of the standard of care is not only the possession of this basic SKEE, but the application of it at the level of the average practitioner of good standing, in the same (school, class, specialty), within the same or similar community, and under the same or similar circumstances. The final element is that the practitioner will use his or her best judgment when ministering to his patients or performing his professional duties.

Although many states still have a form of locality rule for general practitioners, the trend is for specialists to be held to a national standard of care. A District of Columbia case [15] articulated the principles that experts would be required to testify to when advocating that the standard of care was national as opposes to local. They were

1. The standard of care must focus on the course of action that a reasonably prudent doctor in the defendant's specialty would have taken under the same or similar circumstances.
2. The course of action promulgated must be followed nationally.
3. The fact that local doctors may or may not adhere to a national standard is insufficient in and of itself to establish a national standard.
4. In demonstrating that a particular course of action is followed nationally, reference to a published standard, while not required, may be important.
5. Discussions with doctors outside of a particular jurisdiction who agree with the course of action or treatment, at seminars and conventions; or, reference to specific medical literature supporting the course of action or treatment, may be sufficient.
6. An expert's personal opinion does not constitute an affirmation of a national standard of care; thus a statement of what the expert would do under similar circumstances, by itself, is inadequate.
7. National standard of care testimony may not be based upon mere speculation or conjecture.

Geography aside, states such as Massachusetts define the "community in which one practices" as the profession itself [16]. In addition, Massachusetts, like many other states, requires the plaintiff to produce expert testimony to establish standard of care and causation questions, unless these issues are very obvious and are of the type that can easily be understood by a lay person [17].

Differing standards between generalists and specialists

Because the laws vary among the States, there are arguably, depending upon the jurisdiction in which one practices, two standards of care: one for generalists and one for specialists. As a general rule, general practitioners have a greater chance of being held to a standard of care based on what is done in a certain locality, whereas specialists will generally be held more often to a national standard of care. Obviously an expert witness testifying for either side must familiarize himself with the applicable standards, because many experts are from out of state. One slight nuance is the standard of care for those in training programs. In Pennsylvania for instance, there are three standards. The first is for a general practitioner, the second would apply to a resident in a specialty training program, and the third would apply to the specialist. The court in the applicable case [18] noted

> To require a resident to meet the same standard of care as a fully trained specialist would be unrealistic. A resident may have had only days or weeks

of training in the specialized training program ... . If we were to require the resident to exercise the same degree of skill and training as the specialist, we would, in effect, be requiring the resident to do the impossible.

Conversely, in the teaching environment, both the hospital and the supervising attending physicians are responsible for ensuring that the care rendered by a resident conforms to the standard of care governing that particular jurisdiction [19]. Again, it is important for the expert to familiarize himself with the laws of the particular jurisdiction in which he finds himself.

A tangential issue is what standard of care is a general practitioner held to when performing specialty procedures? Again, states vary in their response to this query, and the expert who plans to testify in a given state should know what the standard of care is in that jurisdiction regarding this issue. A Kansas case [20] provides some insight into this question. The court stated

> The trial court noted that a "general practitioner ordinarily doesn't have the skill and knowledge of a specialist." The trial court ultimately concluded, and correctly, by instructing the jury that the defendant in this case held himself out to the public as a general practitioner in dentistry and as such had the duty to use reasonable care and skill for the safety and well-being of the plaintiff. However, when the defendant undertook to perform the work of a specialist he had the duty to use the skill and care of the specialist.
>
> It is the generally accepted rule that a physician or surgeon or dentist who holds himself out to be a specialist is bound to bring to the discharge of his professional duties as a specialist that degree of skill, care and learning ordinarily possessed by specialists of a similar class, having regard to the existing state of knowledge in medicine, surgery and dentistry, that is, a higher degree of skill, care and learning than that of the average practitioner.

Different schools of thought

What about all of those times when there may be several diagnoses that fit the patient's symptoms, or several treatment alternatives for the same condition? Is one liable for choosing the wrong one? How and by whom is this handled? It may all come down to the proverbial war between the experts. A Connecticut case [21] sheds some light on this issue. After the plaintiff presents his case, the defendant has the opportunity to respond, and he is in no different a position than anyone responding to a claim that malpractice was committed. At this point, the defendant offers credible expert evidence that his conduct was acceptable within the profession and hopes that the jury will be persuaded. The court went on to note that

> It is true that an instruction on alternative acceptable methods may tempt jurors to decide that both sets of experts are right, instead of forcing them

to make a difficult choice between opposing experts. The difficulties faced by lay jurors when evaluating expert evidence are, however, endemic to our system of trial by jury. We presume that the jury will abide by its duty to make a thoughtful reasoned decision, applying its common sense and logic to the evidence presented.

A Wisconsin court addressing the same issue stated in its opinion [22]

> If you find that more than one method of treatment ... is recognized, then the [defendant] was at liberty to select any of the recognized methods. The [defendant] was not negligent merely because he made a choice of a recognized alternative method of treatment if he used the required care, skill, and judgment in administering the method. This is true even though other medical witnesses may not agree with him on the choice that was made.

In reality, it may not be the expert with the highest credentials whom the jury chooses to believe. Instead it sometimes becomes a subjective decision based on the ability of an expert to "speak the juror's language." Courts are not immune to this conundrum, and often instruct the jury in the following manner:

> You are not bound by an expert's opinion. In resolving conflicts in expert testimony, weigh the different expert opinions against each other and consider the relative qualifications and credibility of the experts, the reasons and facts supporting their opinions, and whether the facts and reasons given are based on facts you find are established by the evidence in this case [21].

Can experts in one area testify about other areas?

Another thorny issue is crossover testimony. This concerns an expert with a background in one area of medicine testifying in a case dealing with another specialty or subspecialty. Examples of this are chiropractors testifying against orthopedists; ear, nose, and throat physicians testifying against plastic surgeons; general dentists testifying against orthodontists; and so on. The bottom line is that there are three factors to consider when attempting to qualify an expert. The first is whether or not the subject matter is the type that requires expert testimony to aid the trier of fact in rendering its decision. The second is whether or not the area of so called expertise has been scientifically established, so that a valid opinion can be produced by experts in the area. And finally, the court must determine whether or not the witness has the qualifications to render expert testimony on the subject matter. An Idaho court [23] succinctly summarized the position taken by a majority of jurisdictions when it stated

> The witness must demonstrate a knowledge acquired from experience or study of the standards of the specialty of the defendant physician sufficient to enable him to give an expert opinion as to the conformity of the

defendant's conduct to those particular standards, and not to the standards of the witness' particular specialty if it differs from that of the defendant. It is the scope of the witness' knowledge and not the artificial classification by title that should govern the threshold question of admissibility.

The professional witness

Experts don't have an easy job regardless of which side they advocate for. There are reams of records to review and countless consultations with the attorney who has hired you. There is also the wrath of one's brethren that one receives subsequent to deciding to testify against one of his colleagues, particularly if the defendant has a high profile within the field. We have all heard experts referred to as hired guns. The reality is that both sides have their gunslingers, and OK Corral shootouts occur more often than one thinks. Does it create a bias on the part of an expert that 20% or more of his yearly income is derived from giving expert testimony? Can this point be exploited at trial by the opposing side? A Maryland court [24] took this issue head on and noted from an historical perspective that as far back as 1858 jurists lamented

> Perhaps testimony which least deserves credit with a jury is that of skilled witnesses. These gentlemen are usually required to speak, not to the facts, but to opinions; and when this is the case, it is often quite surprising to see with what facility, and to what an extent, their views can be made to correspond with the wishes or the interests of the parties who call them.

In an 1893 address to the New Hampshire Medical Society, Professor Charles Himes noted that expert witnesses

> " … are selected on account of their ability to express a favorable opinion, which, there is great reason to believe, is in many instances the result alone of employment and the bias growing out if it" [25].

In order to expose such bias, a Maryland court [24] noted that experts, especially professional ones, need to be vigorously cross examined about such things as

How much are they being paid for their services regarding the case at hand?
How often do they provide expert testimony in similar types of cases?
Does the witness usually represent the plaintiff or the defendant?
Is the witness often employed by the same attorney?
How much income per year is derived from providing expert testimony?
What percentage of the expert's gross income comes from expert testimony?

Although one would think that this type of questioning would be sufficient to make many potential experts think twice before accepting an invitation to be an expert witness in a case, the court was quick to note that it is not permissible for courts to authorize or tolerate wholesale harassment of expert witnesses by allowing fishing expeditions into their personal and professional financial affairs; such inquiries must be tightly controlled. The court was also adamant about the fact that although an expert witness may devote a significant portion of his time to forensic testimony, and reap a substantial amount of income from doing so, this fact does not in and of itself mean that the testimony he provides is not honest, accurate, and credible. It is up to the jury to weigh these questions and determine the extent of any bias.

Dealing with the unscrupulous expert

So how do we deal with the unscrupulous expert? Read the following excerpt [26]:

> Some years ago one of us had the occasion to attend ... a medical malpractice suit filed in New York City. Like other suits, this one attacked the professional integrity of a practicing physician, impugning a 35 year medical career. ... [T]he plaintiff's attorney ... called an expert medical witness to testify under oath that in his opinion this physician had practiced medicine below the prevailing standard of care.
>
> On the surface ... this expert witness may have seemed an impressive figure. He testified that he was a member of a department of Head and Neck Surgery at a hospital in a Manhattan and a professor at a medical school. He proceeded to offer opinions about the way in which the surgical procedure in question should have been performed, and justified his views by displaying anatomical diagrams which appeared to come from standard textbooks. Under [cross examination] ... it emerged that he had never actually performed the procedure at issue. In fact he was not a surgeon, or a medical school professor. He also admitted that part of his testimony involved the use of altered anatomic diagrams.
>
> ... Though the expert ... in this case [was] thoroughly discredited during the cross examination neither he nor the attorney who hired him were seriously at risk of any professional discipline. This case might have been lost if not ... for a friend ... who recognized the expert witness as ... a fraud.

Although not a daily occurrence, the harrowing scenario depicted above does repeat itself every now and then. In 1998 The Hillsborough County Medical Society (Florida) thought enough of this issue to develop an Expert Witness Committee (EWC). This committee is charged with evaluating claims of misconduct by expert witnesses and making subsequent recommendations to the disciplinary body of the governing association based on their findings. The following outlines the general guidelines that physicians who wish to testify as expert witnesses in Florida must follow [27]:

1. The physician should have current experience and ongoing knowledge in the area of clinical medicine about which he is testifying.

2. The physician's review of the medical facts should be thorough, fair, and impartial; and should not exclude any relevant information to create a view that favors either the plaintiff or the defendant.
3. The physician's testimony should reflect an evaluation of performance in light of generally accepted standards.
4. The physician should make a clear distinction between medical malpractice and medical mal-occurrence.
5. The physician should make every effort to assess the relationship of the alleged substandard practice to the outcome, since deviation from a practice standard is not always causally related to a bad outcome.
6. The physician should be willing to subject transcripts of deposition and courtroom testimony to peer review.

These guidelines would apply not only to opinions rendered in malpractice cases, but also to sworn testimony given at administrative hearings, such as those before a State Board of Medicine or Office of Professional Conduct and the like. The admonitions would also apply to testimony proffered in workman's compensation and disability cases, testimony given in trials stemming from general negligence claims, and even to testimony provided in criminal cases.

In a case [28] dealing with an expert's irresponsible testimony that resulted in his Association membership being suspended, the court stated

> There is a great deal of skepticism about expert evidence. It is well known that expert witnesses are often paid very handsome fees, and common sense suggests that a financial stake can influence expert testimony, especially when it is technical and esoteric and hence difficult to refute in terms intelligible to judges and jurors. More policing of expert witnesses is required, not less. Not that professional self-regulation is wholly trustworthy. Professional associations have their own axes to grind. ... . We note finally that there is a strong national interest ... in identifying and sanctioning poor quality physicians and thereby improving the quality of health care. Although [the expert] did not treat the malpractice plaintiff for whom he testified, his testimony ... was a type of medical service and if the quality of his testimony reflected the quality of his medical judgment, he is probably a poor physician.

Should one be an expert?

Whenever the author gives risk management seminars to dental audiences, I always ask how many in the audience would testify on behalf of a plaintiff against one of their colleagues? Almost no hands go up. I then ask how many in the audience would elect to testify on behalf of one of their colleagues should they be sued? Almost everyone would do so. I then tell them that what they have just exhibited is what is known as a conspiracy of silence. Looking at our legal system, warts and all, I cannot help but compare it to what occurs in other countries worldwide. In many places injured patients have no access to redress, and in other countries it is just plain difficult. Sure, we have our flaws and sometimes we are rightfully accused of having gone over the top, but the bottom line is that this is the system we have, and for the most part it works. An overwhelming majority of malpractice suits against single defendants that go to trial are won by the doctor.

I still say that if I get sued for malpractice, I want one of my peers to tell me "Larry, you made a mistake, time to pay the piper" or I want him or her to say "Listen, what you did was reasonable even if the outcome was less than desirable; I'll be happy to go to bat for you." The bottom line is that this is why I carry malpractice insurance.

Summary

The author hopes that this essay has enlightened the reader to the role that the expert witness plays in our legal system. He provides a valuable service for the trier of fact who must decide issues foreign to the lay person. He has an awesome responsibility, and must literally decide in his own mind that one of his colleagues did or did not conform to the standard of care as practiced within one's field and community, be it local or national. The expert must be willing to undergo intense scrutiny and cross examination at trial; it is not something for the faint of heart to get involved with. By virtue of participating in the legal system, one sometimes becomes a pariah within his profession.

I leave you with this final thought. Every one of us who practices in the healing arts has or will commit malpractice. We do not mean to, but accidents, mistakes, and oversights happen. When that happens and a patient is injured as a result, if you are the defendant, pay the freight. If you are asked to be an expert for the defendant, do it. There may be arguments and rationalizations to explain why whatever it was occurred. This may be enough for the jury to decide on a smaller award. Maybe the plaintiff is asking for the world and should only be entitled to a small country. Whatever it is, if you can help, do so. Finally, if you are called to represent the plaintiff, do it. Simply put, it is the ethical thing to do. We must police ourselves. Society has granted us a license to make a lot of money and have a respected, sometimes exalted, position in the community. Honor that license by helping those in need. After all, we did take an oath to help heal the injured. Hippocrates didn't specify how the injury had to occur.

References

[1] Black's law dictionary. 5th edition. St. Paul (MN): West Publishing Co.; 1979.
[2] Amoco Chemical Corp v Hill, Del. Super., 318 A.2d 614.
[3] Russo v Griffin, 510 A.2d 436, 1986.

[4] Mello v Cohen, 724 A.2d 471, 1998.
[5] Plummer v District of Columbia Bd. Of Funeral Dirs., 730 A.2d 159, 1999.
[6] Jones v Young, 607 N.E.2d 224, 1992.
[7] Reese v Stroh, 907 P.2d 282, 1995.
[8] Weatherford v Glassman, 500 S.E.2d 466, 1998.
[9] Heatherly. Industrial Health Council, 504 S.E.2d 102, 1998.
[10] Brown v McQuinn, 501 So.2d 1093, 1986.
[11] Roberts v Warren, 782 So.2d 717, 2001.
[12] Chapel v Allison, 785 P.2d 204, 1990.
[13] Tenn. Code Ann. Sec. 29-26-115, 1980.
[14] Mccarty v Mladineo, 636 So.2d 377, 1994.
[15] Hawes v Chua, 769 A.2d 797, 2001.
[16] Brune v Belinkoff, 235 N.E.2d 793, 1968.
[17] Pongonis v Saab, 1005 N.E.2d 28, 1985.
[18] Jistarri v Nappi, 549 A.2d 210 (Pa.Super), 1988.
[19] Rouse v Pitt County Memorial Hosp. Inc., 447 S.E.2d 505 (N.C.App.), 1994.
[20] Simpson v Davis, 549 P.2d 950, 1976.
[21] Wasfi v Chaddha, 588 A.2d 204, 1991.
[22] Nowatske v Osterloh, 543 N.W.2d 265, 1996.
[23] Clark v Prenger, 760 P.2d 1182, 1988.
[24] Wrobleski v de Lara, 727 A.2d 930, 1999
[25] 135 J. Franklin Inst., 409, 1893.
[26] Luria, LW, Agliano DS. Abusive expert testimony: toward peer review. Civil Justice Memos. Manhattan Institute. No. 31, April 1997.
[27] Expert witness committee. Articles and guidelines. Hillsborough County Medical Association Inc. Updated May 4, 1998.
[28] Justin v American Association of Neurological Surgeons, 253 F.3d 967, (Ct. App. 7th Cir 2001).

ELSEVIER
SAUNDERS

SURGICAL
CLINICS OF
NORTH AMERICA

Surg Clin N Am 87 (2007) 903–918

A Comprehensive Primer
of Surgical Informed Consent

James W. Jones, MD, PhD[a,*],
Lawrence B. McCullough, PhD[b],
Bruce W. Richman, MA[c]

[a]31 LaCosta Road, Montgomery, TX 77356, USA
[b]Center for Medical Ethics and Health Policy, Baylor College of Medicine,
One Baylor Plaza, Houston, TX 77030, USA
[c]2809 Butterfield Court, Columbia, MO 65203, USA

The clinical skills required in the informed consent process tend not to be taught to fellows, residents, and medical students within the formal curriculum [1]. Furthermore, surgical residents are seldom supervised during their communication with patients. As a result, faculty and trainees alike forego an opportunity to identify, evaluate, and address weaknesses in the resident's interpersonal skills with patients generally, and during the informed consent dialogue in particular. Surgical practice is distinct from nonsurgical medical practice in a number of regards, primarily because of the operation. Surgical therapy occurs as a specific event, usually requiring entry into the patient's body; the therapeutic event can be timed exactly (assigning culpability); the emotional stress on the patient is greater; and the surgical patient plays a more passive role than patients of other medical specialties once anesthesia is induced. The patient then becomes incapable of participatory intraoperative decision-making; and surgeon assumes full control of the decision-making process. Surgeons may consequently have a less fully developed sense of an active physician-patient partnership in the healing process than colleagues in other specialties, and this can affect their approach to informed consent. The surgeon may also assume that the referring physician has already made the necessary intellectual and emotional preparations and effectively has obtained the patient's consent for surgical resolution of the clinical problem. In combination, these factors can lead the unwitting

This article originally appeared in the Thoracic Surgery Clinics, November 2005; Informed Consent: It's Not Just Signing a Form.

 * Corresponding author
 E-mail address: jwjones@bcm.tmc.edu (J.W. Jones).

doi:10.1016/j.suc.2007.07.012
surgical.theclinics.com

surgeon to underestimate the capacity and willingness of the patient to participate in the informed consent process that should precede induction of anesthesia. As a consequence, the surgeon can lose the opportunity to form an effective therapeutic alliance with the patient.

The informed consent process

Historical development

The traditional debate over the requirement that physicians involve patients in therapeutic decisions was transformed by the ethical and legal analysis of several important legal cases involving surgical treatment. The starting point is the common law of informed consent as a patient's right, a twentieth century concept. Two key features of the legal history of informed consent are relevant here: simple consent and informed consent.

Simple consent involves one question: "Did the patient agree to be treated"? If the answer is yes, then the conditions of consent are thought to be satisfied. If the answer is no, then the conditions are not satisfied and the surgeon cannot operate.

In 1914, Judge Benjamin Cardozo wrote a landmark opinion in the case *Schloendorff v The Society of New York Hospital*, which legally defined simple consent and changed the history of American medical ethics [2]. Cardozo wrote that, "every human being of adult years and sound mind has a right to determine what shall be done with his body; and a surgeon who performs an operation without his patient's consent commits an assault, for which he is liable in damages, ... except in cases of emergency, where the patient is unconscious, and where it is necessary to operate before consent can be obtained" [2]. The patient's autonomy was at least equally important. Respect for autonomy obligates the physician to seek for the patient the greater balance of goods over harms, as those goods and harms are understood and balanced from the patient's perspective. The surgeon no longer possessed authority to act unilaterally on clinical judgments.

Although many surgeons today practice as though simple consent is still the ethical standard, the subsequent legal history of informed consent focused on the nature and quality of the physician's disclosure and obligation. Instead of one question, two questions must be asked: "Did the physician provide the patient with an adequate amount of information?", and "On the basis of this information, did the patient consent?" As the common law developed from the late 1950s through the early 1970s, two standards of adequacy emerged. The first is the professional community or professional practice standard [3,4]. Under this physician-oriented standard of disclosure, the patient should be told what an appropriately experienced physician in the community would tell the patient about the patient's condition, alternatives available for managing the condition, and generalize the benefits and risks of each alternative.

The courts gradually came to regard the professional community standard as inadequate, largely because of growing skepticism about the integrity of a solely physician-based standard. A major event in the development of an alternative standard was the case of *Canterbury v Spence*, decided in 1972 but occurring in 1958 [5]. This court rejected the professional community standard as inadequate and replaced it with the reasonable person standard. Informed consent involves meeting the needs of the "reasonable patient." This legal construct means that the informational needs of a patient should be identified on the basis of what a reasonable patient, not a particular patient in a particular, subjective circumstance, needs to know to make a meaningful decision. The patient needs to know material information (ie, what the nonprofessional patient is unlikely to encounter in daily life). The discussion need not be a disquisition, and surely the physician is not compelled to give his or her patient a short medical education; the disclosure role summons the physician only to a reasonable explanation. This means generally informing the patient in nontechnical terms what is at stake.

Patients may need, and often welcome, an offer to help think through their options. Because the decisions often involve subtle tradeoffs that are best understood and judged only by the patient, the surgeon should monitor himself or herself against coercing the patient, overtly or subtly. He or she may, and should, present the best case for surgical treatment if it is professionally considered to be the safest and most effective course, but the detriments of other alternatives or the benefits of surgery should not be exaggerated. In explaining the risks and discomforts attendant to any course, surgeons should be wary of making these sound so frightening that the patient rejects all varieties of crucial treatment.

In addition to the obligation to obtain consent or refusal, the patient's "yes" or "no" to intervention, the reasonable person standard includes a duty to explain clinical judgments and recommendations that enable the patient to make an independent, informed decision. The patient's perspective of his or her own interests should be respected by the surgeon. The ethical principle of respect for autonomy captures what is at stake clinically. The surgeon should acknowledge and accept the integrity of the competent patient's values and beliefs, whether or not the surgeon agrees with them, and should provide the patient with an adequate amount of information. A physician's disclosure is adequate when it includes the salient features of the physician's clinical thinking in arriving at the recommended therapy and explains to the patient the basic thought process that brought the surgeon to the conclusion that surgical management is a reasonable course of therapeutic action for this patient in this case [1].

The process

Surgeons should conceptualize and practice informed consent as a continuing process, rather than as a static event. Properly used, informed consent provides the basis for a strong and enduring professional alliance between the surgeon and patient, with shared responsibility for decision making [4]. Thus understood, informed consent is not simply the signature on the authorization form. This is legal documentation, and whereas documentation is important in satisfying the legal component of the consent process, documentation does not constitute the most important ethical element of informed consent. The patient's signature on the informed consent form is far less crucial than the process that it serves to document.

The concept of informed consent includes three elements, each of which presumes and builds on its predecessor [4]. The first is disclosure by the surgeon to the patient of adequate clear information about the patient's diagnosis; the alternatives available to treat the patient's problem, including surgical and nonsurgical management; the benefits and risks of each alternative, including nonintervention (ie, allowing the natural history of the disease to continue); and a frank explanation of those factors about which the medical profession, and the individual surgeon in particular, are uncertain and cannot provide guarantees. This disclosure should be individually tailored in its presentation to the intellectual and emotional capacity of each patient to understand, absorb, and retain information and make decisions. The second of the three elements is the patient's understanding of this clinical information. The third element is the patient's process of decision, based not only on what the surgeon has told them, but information they have been exposed to from other sources, including other physicians, family and friends, and perhaps an acquaintance who has had a similar procedure; what they have read by independently researching the problem; and their own emotional response to illness and all that it changes in one's life. The ethical requirements of each of these three elements are now considered in greater clinical detail.

Disclosure obligations

No surgeon wants to be sued, lose patients' confidence, or undergo the humiliation of admitting errors; all are among the distinct dangers of full disclosure. The spirit of informed consent, however, has ethically and legally replaced paternalism in surgery. Informed consent does not stop with the agreement to accept therapy [6]. Mutual decision-making by the physician and patient (or family, when the patient agrees or cannot participate) about treatment has the same ethical obligations throughout the course of therapy.

Kantian ethics suggest that although one must avoid deception, truth may be selectively told. Selective truth telling is the way personal lives are lived; one chooses to whom one discloses information or not, and the sensitivity or completeness of information disclosed. This ethical axiom does not apply in the surgeon-patient relationship concerning specifics of the patient's condition and therapy. The physician must help the patient to understand both what is planned preoperatively and how treatment is proceeding.

The extent of disclosure is generally based on the physician's identification of information that should influence diagnosis, treatment planning, and outcomes. This includes knowledge that the average layperson cannot be expected to have, but needs to know to participate meaningfully in treatment decisions and planning for the future.

The patient's understanding

McKneally and Martin [7] examined the consent process before major surgery from the patient's perspective. Several recurrent themes of patient's mental processes were learned: a belief in surgical cure, enhancement of trust through the referral process, idealization of the specialist surgeon, belief in expertise rather than medical information, resignation to risks of treatment, and acceptance of an expert recommendation as consent to treatment. Those patients with serious illnesses, being sent to a specific surgeon or a specific institution, had already firmly committed to operative therapy and the consent process was a formality. Patients constructed their belief systems through faith before the informed consent process took place. Informed consent in surgical practice must respond to these ethical challenges and opportunities. The surgeon should consider informed consent as an ethically essential course of action that can be used to strengthen the surgeon-patient alliance with mutual benefits. Although surgeons hesitate to mention it and its real effect is unquantified, there is a noteworthy placebo effect in surgery [8] that should not be overlooked.

Apart from legal considerations that are minimal by professional moral standards, surgeons must always remember that having major surgery is one of the most stressful and fearful events of patients' lives. The law emphasizes the physician's role in the informed consent process. This is not surprising; patients bring tort actions against the physicians, not vice versa. The courts have not been asked to address the patient's role in the informed consent process. Ethics addresses both the physician's and the patient's roles and responsibilities in the informed consent transaction. Ethical consideration goes on to evaluate what the surgeon has explained and what the patient has understood, the second substantive element in informed consent. Patients need to understand what surgeons tell them about a proposed surgical procedure.

More substantively, patients need to understand that they are being asked to authorize surgical management. Faden and Beauchamp [4] point out that this means that the patient must understand that by consenting to surgical management the patient authorizes the surgeon and surgical team to perform the procedure that the surgeon has described to the patient. The patient must also understand that the surgery cannot proceed without the patient's permission.

Finally, the patient should understand what is being authorized [4,9]. The patient needs to grasp the nature of the procedure, its goals, its expected duration, and what can be expected during the near- and long-term recovery process. Sequelae of surgery, particularly functional changes that affect job performance, valued activities, or sexuality, and aesthetic changes, such as the length and appearance of scar tissue, must be understood.

Documentation in the medical record

A well-crafted note in the medical record can be a valuable clinical aid to the surgeon, as a checklist and record of the information exchanged. The consent note should include a listing of the people in attendance, the description of the procedure in lay terms, the goal of the procedure as described (with any figures about failure rates), the major aspects or steps of the procedure that were discussed, the benefits and risks of the procedure which were discussed and the pertinent questions asked, as well as expectations for the course of both near- and long-term recovery. The note should specify that the patient authorizes the surgeon and surgical team to perform the procedure. The contents of the note can be reviewed with the patient and the patient encouraged to identify what is still unclear or confusing, so that these matters can be addressed.

The process of deciding

Patient's psychology during consent

McKneally and Martin [7] found that many patients have already determined the absolute necessity of surgical therapy before seeing the surgeon and are focused on obtaining operations; the informed consent process should both supply the necessary information and serve to qualify the patient's belief system.

The process of making an explicit decision by the patient on the surgeon's recommendation is importantly placed as the third and culminating element of the informed consent process. In making their decisions about surgery, patients should appreciate that present conditions and actions have future consequences. The patient should be able to reason from present events to future consequences and have an adequately developed sense of the probabilities that these projected outcomes, called cognitive understanding, may indeed occur. The surgeon's important role in the development of cognitive understanding includes correcting errors in the patient's information, helping to augment the patient's fund of knowledge, and helping patients grasp the nature and likelihood of the future consequences attendant on each of the therapeutic choices available to them.

In response to patients who desire only a small role in the decision-making process but want surgical management of their problem, the surgeon should nonetheless provide an explanation of the surgical procedure by reviewing the major issues, such as contents of the consent form. The surgeon should also prepare the patient for the immediate postoperative period with a brief explanation of what this entails so that the patient is not surprised or alarmed when they wake up in the recovery area or surgical intensive care unit.

Patients considering surgery should also evaluate benefits and risks of the alternatives available to them. These are value judgments and concern how much worth to attach to potential favorable and unfavorable outcomes associated with each available option. Making such value judgments involves evaluative understanding, a clinical consideration overlooked altogether in the law governing informed consent. In making decisions about surgery, each patient needs to make value judgments about the benefits, risks, and discomforts of surgery; of other available medical interventions; and whether surgery or other invention is less dire than living with the risks and discomforts of untreated illness. Evaluative understanding is just as essential to the patient's decision-making as cognitive understanding.

The surgeon can help the patient to develop evaluative understanding of available alternatives. Asking a patient, "What is important to you as you consider ....," with the ellipsis completed with each alternative, is effective in eliciting the patient's values [10]. The surgeon should discern patterns of values in conversation with the patient and identify them for patients who are struggling to articulate what is important to them. Patients do not make decisions on the basis of isolated values, and helping patients to connect otherwise unarticulated concerns promotes individual autonomy. They might consider job performance, sexual activity, mental function, physical appearance, and, particularly important, hobbies of the retired to define their values. For example, it does not respect the values of a patient who is an avid hunter to place a pacemaker on the side of the chest from which the patient fires a shotgun while dove hunting. Such assistance also directs the surgeon's relationship to the patient's most fundamental values and beliefs because they give meaning to the alternative possible futures the patient must contemplate. Evaluative understanding is the area that may depart most radically from the surgeon's own value system, requiring a nondirective approach. Once the patient has identified his or her relevant values and evaluated the alternatives on this basis, it is time for the surgeon to offer a recommendation.

The patient should not only feel free to ask questions, but should be encouraged to do so. The meaning of questions from the patient and the patient's family is not always readily apparent. The first question of many patients is often, "How long will this operation take?", and the surgeon should respond with an estimate of the customary range of time it has taken them to complete this procedure in the past. The surgeon should also understand that the real question being asked usually is, "When should my family begin to worry that things aren't going well?". To help patients with questions they have difficulty articulating, the surgeon may direct the conversation to questions that earlier patients have asked about this procedure, and invite the patient to discuss these questions in the context of their personal concerns. Patients usually become relaxed enough to start asking their own questions and genuinely begin to seek information about the operation.

Respect for the autonomy of the patient means that the patient's decision should be free of substantially controlling influences [4,11]. The physician should make a recommendation only after the patient has developed evaluative understanding without fear of bringing undue influence to bear on the patient's autonomy. Most patients highly value the surgeon's recommendation as they struggle to reach their own decisions. Appropriately timed recommendations play an important role in the informed consent process, and may even support the independent nature of the patient's decision.

The ethics of the informed consent process emphasizes the role of this process in developing solid rapport with the patient. Such a rapport has a number of clinical advantages. First, the surgeon does not function as a disinterested and unbiased source of information, consulted as one might consult a book as a noninteractive source. Instead, the surgeon has important experiences and opinions with which to assist the patient in the decision-making process, not the least important of which are the technical information and knowledge of the patient's personal medical history. Failure by surgeons to provide patients with the full range of their knowledge for fear of violating a patient's autonomy could mean that the patient does not become genuinely informed, and ultimately defeats the high-minded principle the surgeon is seeking to protect the patient. Ultimately, no one knows more or is more intimately concerned about the details of the patient's surgical treatment than the surgeon and the patient, which makes their mutually respectful cooperation essential to the process of genuine informed consent. Second, forming a therapeutic alliance with the patient through the informed consent process results in a more informed, prepared patient, who has developed a sense of individual responsibility in the transaction. Patient compliance may increase, leading to a smoother, more effective postoperative course. In an era of managed care, this outcome helps to promote the valued goal of the more economically efficient use of expensive medical resources, like surgery. Third, the open and honest two-way communication called for by the ethics of the informed consent process should increase the patient's confidence and trust in the surgeon. This goes a long way toward establishing good rapport with patients, and advance the value of surgery for both surgeon and patient.

Definition of the process

Formed by this ethical analysis, the informed consent process becomes a process of mutual decision-making. The surgeon and the patient both have active and important roles in this process, and responsibilities to discharge. The surgeon, as the patient's fiduciary, should share beneficence-based clinical judgment with the patient. As the patient's fiduciary (ie, as someone who acts primarily to protect the patient's interests), the surgeon should also be committed to doing the right thing for the patient, but the ultimate decision about what is right for the patient rests with the patient. For this reason, the ethics of the informed consent process places strong emphasis on the surgeon's respect for the patient's autonomy.

Initiation of the consent process in the surgical holding area just before the operation is scheduled to begin should be avoided in all but the most urgent or most minor procedures. Instead, the discussion should be initiated well in advance of surgery because decisions should be made without added tension and with the time necessary to a major life decision. Outpatient visits for preoperative work-up provide an ideal opportunity to conduct the informed consent process.

Extent of the surgeon's influence

The surgeon's recommendations have a proper role in the informed consent process. Most patients value their surgeon's recommendations and customarily give them considerable weight in their own decision-making process about whether to accept surgical management of their condition. In principle, surgeons exercise permissible influence through their recommendations.

Altering the frame of reference to influence the patient's decision by excessively emphasizing either benefits or risks, a process termed "framing" [1], poses clinical ethical challenges. Framing is inconsistent with both the surgeon's fiduciary role and with respect for patient autonomy, and should be avoided. For example, the surgeon may describe surgical risks as merely routine, as they may seem to the surgeon, and the benefits as certain. These descriptions may be consistent with the individual surgeon's experience, but they are incorrect in terms of predicting the outcome for the specific operative patient and are deceptive. Inadvertently, a surgeon may seek to reassure a patient by making such statements as "I cannot remember the last time we lost a patient from this operation." Framing in this manner before the patient decides to have surgery is ethically questionable, because the characterization can discourage development of the patient's own critical evaluation.

Surgeons should also avoid a particularly corrupt and common type of framing commonly termed "crepe hanging." This involves exaggerating the gravity of the patient's situation, and of the operation, to increase the patient's estimation of and gratitude toward the surgeon when things go well, as they were expected to by the surgeon in the first place. Should the surgery have a poor outcome, the surgeon has only to say that this is as he predicted and the patient nevertheless agreed to proceed.

Surgeons should be especially aware of subtle framing effects that can occur when substituting descriptive terms for quantitative terms, especially in the characterization of risks. For example, the surgeon might tell the patient facing surgery for glaucoma, "You will lose your eyesight without the procedure." The more truthful statement, however, is that a certain percentage of people in this circumstance, perhaps 15% in this hypothetical case, lose eyesight without the corrective procedure. Surgeons should adhere to quantitative descriptions whenever possible in the early steps of the informed consent process and then help the patient to evaluate this information in the steps concerned with cognitive and evaluative understanding.

Special circumstances during informed consent

Conflicting professional opinions

Patients occasionally encounter conflicting opinions among surgeons or between the referring physician and the referral surgeon. Everyone in the medical profession understands, but may not readily acknowledge, that clinical judgment can vary widely among the specialties and even among practitioners within the same specialty. For example, the referring physician may focus on the operation's morbidity risks, whereas the surgeon may be most concerned about reducing disease-related mortality and so may discount, to some extent, the inconvenience, cost, morbidity, and discomfort of the procedure [12]. The guiding principle when differences of judgment occur was articulated two centuries ago by the Scottish physician John Gregory (1724–1773). He emphasized that the surgeons and physicians should manage such disagreements with a view always toward protecting the interests of the patient [12].

Consent with multiple physicians

The typical surgical patient receives ongoing care from physicians in several specialties, including surgery, before, during, and after procedures. The tendency exists in these team contexts to assume that others have already spoken with the patient, have explained what is happening, and have taken the patient through the informed consent process. This assumption can lead to a defective informed consent process, especially regarding the surgical procedure being contemplated. The operating surgeon should take a preventive ethics approach to this potential problem by accepting responsibility for taking the patient through the consent process for the operation. The anesthesiologist should participate in this process with reference to the alternatives, benefits, and effects of anesthesia options. All physicians, especially those in training, should avoid giving answers to questions outside their specialty and about which they are uncertain, and avoid areas apart from their expertise.

When multiple surgeons are involved, the surgical specialist who performs the most essential and most complication-prone parts of the operation has the greatest responsibility regarding informed consent. This physician should tell the patient who the other participants are and what their roles will be in the patient's care. This preventive ethics approach minimizes the chance that the patient will become confused or concerned about the involvement of multiple surgeons.

Patients who are undecided or refuse surgery

Some patients may refuse surgical intervention after an adequate informed consent process because they are in a state of indecision. If the consent process has gone well, this indecision usually results from a patient's ambivalence over similarly attractive alternatives. The patient may often also be frightened about having an operation and understandably may resolve indecision in favor of nonsurgical management of the condition.

In this case the surgeon should explain that the patient has caused no offense by being undecided. Such a decision, after all, does not preclude a decision for surgery later. In elective surgeries, the patient should be encouraged to think matters through and to determine if the decision will become more apparent with time. The surgeon should explain, however, that the postponement of surgical treatment, as cases of cancers, for example, may change the nature of benefits and risks. If the surgeon decides to remain on such a patient's case, the patient should be so informed, and told that the surgeon will discuss the patient's decision at any time. The canons of medical ethics and common courtesy are violated if the surgeon vocalizes disappointment, anger, or threatens to refuse future treatment toward the patient for not affirming trust in the consulting surgeon.

A patient's refusal to have surgery is not itself evidence of the patient's diminished decision-making capacity. Nonetheless, refusal when surgery is clearly indicated does raise a "red flag" and prompts any thoughtful surgeon to question the patient's decision-making capacity, especially in potentially life-threatening circumstances. A patient who refuses such surgery without attaching importance to mortality, morbidity, or reduced quality of life causes a surgeon frustration and concern. Recent studies of noncompliance confirm that failure in communication can result in patient refusal of the physician's recommendation, or noncooperation with a treatment plan [13].

The surgeon's first response to refusal of surgery should be to review with the patient his or her understanding of the condition, the nature of the surgical procedure, and its benefits and risks. The patient's cognitive understanding may be incomplete, and the patient may reconsider when more complete understanding has been developed. The surgeon's second response should be to explore the patient's evaluative understanding. Of particular concern should be possible mistrust of physicians (perhaps based on some prior experience); pressing obligations; or emotional factors like anxiety, depression, or fear. The surgeon's third response should be to acknowledge value conflicts when they occur, and work with the patient to identify a management plan that accords with the patient's values. If the surgeon believes that the patient's values are supported by surgery, the surgeon should point this out and ask the patient to reconsider. The preventive ethics approach to refusal of surgery should be respectful exploration of the patient's reasoning, on the assumption that patients, by their own lights, have good reasons for refusal but may, with additional information and reflection, reconsider and accept surgery. Surgeons should not assume that the patient's competence is somehow diminished or compromised just because he withholds consent.

One very helpful response to refusals when surgery's value in averting mortality is unclear is to offer the patient the alternative of a trial of nonsurgical management. Nonsurgical management may be supported by patient values that emerge during the consent process. The patient should be informed of this possibility and a mutual plan developed to monitor the nonsurgical trial of management. The goal should be to identify mutually acceptable criteria for evaluating the nonsurgical management and for reconsidering it. Should a patient be disinclined to accept surgery or any other invasive management as the first option, the surgeon could propose a trial of medical management and agree with the patient on the conditions under which the surgeon initiates surgical intervention. Such circumstances could include recurrent and worsening pathology, even on a regular schedule of medication, unacceptable side effects of medication, or increasing risk of mortality.

Problems with the patient's decision-making capacity

Some patients may still experience difficulty making decisions, regardless of how ethically, astutely, and carefully the surgeon has attended to the informed consent process. The hospital's consultation-liaison psychiatrist, a physician who has the expertise to evaluate patients' decision-making capacity, can be a valuable advisor and ally. The patient should be told of the role of the psychiatrist to the extent that this is possible. The surgeon should make the following request. First, the psychiatrist should evaluate the patient for a formal cognitive or objective disorder or other psychiatric disturbance that might significantly affect the patient's ability to make decisions, and then determine whether the condition is susceptible to treatment. Second, the psychiatrist and the surgeon should agree on a clear delineation of boundaries in their treatment of the patient. Each should understand what the other will do to restore the patient's decision-making capacity and cooperate with one another. Third, the psychiatrist and surgeon should develop a plan for improving the patient's decision-making capacity so that the patient is able to participate in the informed consent process. In all cases, the surgeon should not use consultation-liaison psychiatry simply to declare a patient incompetent [13], thereby enabling others to make decisions for the patient, or discharging the patient to the management of other specialties. Patients with waxing and waning decisional capacity often experience periods of lucidity, and may choose to provide informed consent for surgery during such a period, specifying that statements they may subsequently make while confused should not supersede decisions made during a period of lucidity. These have been called "Ulysses contracts" in the bioethics literature [1,14].

Surrogate decisions

Working up the patient who exhibits problems with decision-making capacity with the aid of consultation-liaison psychiatry should lead to the reliable identification of patients who have irreversibly lost the capacity to participate in the decision-making process. By common law and now in many states by statutory law, family members are asked to make decisions for such patients [15]. There is a stable consensus in the bioethics literature for how this process should occur [14].

Family members should not be asked, "What would you do?" or "What do you want to do?", because these questions invite family members inadvertently to mix up their own concerns and values with those of the patient. Family members should be asked what they believe is important to the patient at this time and in these circumstances. The goal is to try to construct what the patient's evaluative understanding is as closely as possible. On this basis, the remaining steps of the consent process should be completed. This leads to what is known as "substituted judgment" [14].

Sometimes, for a variety of reasons, family members cannot achieve substituted judgment. In such cases they should be asked to make the decision that in their view protects and promotes their loved one's interests. The best way to assist family members in these circumstances is to encourage patients to take a preventive ethics approach on their own. All patients in their geriatric years, those with chronic diseases, and those in the early stages of dementia should be encouraged to express their values and preferences in advance. Advance directives have legal standing in most states.

Surrogate decisions that inaccurately represent the patient's wishes are not ethically binding on the surgeon, provided the surgeon has a basis for reasonable certainty that the surrogate is mistaken before acting contrary to the surrogate's instructions [14]. When the disputed decision is important enough, the court can be petitioned for appointment of a conservator. Surrogate decision-making fails to reflect the patient's wishes accurately in 70% of important treatment issues [16]. If the surgeon chooses to override the faulty surrogate decision when the surrogate is otherwise entitled to control an important decision, surgeon-family conflicts are likely. It is wise to notify the institutional ethics committee or chief of staff in such cases.

Pediatric consent

As a matter of law, parents are in authority over their minor children and are empowered to engage in the informed consent process on their child's behalf. Minor children, however, are not mere objects; they have their own values and preferences for how they want to receive health care. The American Academy of Pediatrics supports the view that children should participate in decision-making commensurate with their developmental capacity [17]. Pediatric surgeons confront conceptual and clinical challenges regarding pediatric assent. Adolescent patients, particularly those with chronic diseases about which the patient has become quite knowledgeable and mature, may be able to complete the steps of the informed consent process as well as adults. When this is the case, the patient's autonomy should be respected by the surgeon and by the adolescent's parents. In these circumstances the surgeon's responsibilities include pointing out to the parents that their child is capable of making an adult decision that deserves respect. When there are differences between parent and child, the surgeon should offer his or her services as a good-faith negotiator. The goal should be to reach a commonly accepted decision rather than to decide whose decision wins.

Not all adolescents can complete the informed consent process, nor can younger children. Nonetheless, children are capable of understanding to a degree appropriate to their age and emotional development that they have a disease, what parts of the body the disease involves, and that surgery can help. These matters should be explained to the patient, when the goal is not so much to obtain the patient's consent as to provide information about the clinical course to which the patient's parents have already consented. This concept has led to such practices as familiarizing children with the hospital, including operative and postoperative areas, before elective surgery.

When supervised trainees do the surgery

The medical profession has an ethical and social obligation to educate physicians and surgeons to meet the needs of future generations of patients. The first teaching hospitals in America were modeled on the British infirmaries and funded from public and private sources. These hospitals provided free care to the poor, and were seen by academic physicians as training sites where a presumed sense of reciprocity obligates indigent patients to serve willingly as teaching material in exchange for their care [18]. This assumption is now considered incompatible with the process of informed consent, which is understood to include the patient's awareness and agreement that trainees may participate in the treatment process. The American Medical Association Council on Ethical and Judicial Affairs has established a clear position on the relationship between patients and trainees on clinical rotations: "Patients should be informed of the identity and training status of individuals involved in their care, and all health care professionals share the responsibility for properly identifying themselves" [19]. Before patients can accept the role of teaching subject, they must be made aware that they have been offered the part.

Informed consent in research

Some ethical constructs, particularly those involving informed consent and the conduct of research, have been so uniformly accepted as necessary to the rights of patients and the integrity of scientific method that they have been codified into international declarations and federal law. Sade [20] summarized the various historical proclamations and their ethical implications in scientific publication. Once surgery embarks into research, surgical autonomy has compelling ethical limits. When the selection process for a medication, graft, or implant is randomized or preassigned, when the choice is not primarily determined or influenced by the patient's individual clinical characteristics, or when the clinical outcome cannot be predicted and alternatives exist, the procedure must be considered clinical research rather than clinical care, and the laws, customs, restrictions, and ethical considerations specific to research become applicable. Surgeons must modify their own behavior accordingly, and observe the legal and ethical conventions that ensure integrity of scientific investigation and the safety of research subjects. Institutional approval must be sought and received before initiation of a research study to ensure the soundness of the science and the safety of patients.

References

[1] McCullough L, Jones JW, Brody BA. Informed consent: autonomous decision making of the surgical patient. In: McCullough LB, Jones JW, Brody BA, editors. Surgical ethics. New York: Oxford University Press; 1998.

[2] *Schloendorff v Society of New York Hospital*, 211 NY 125, 126, 105 NE 92, (1914).

[3] Wear S. Enhancing clinician provision of informed consent and counseling: some pedagogical strategies. J Med Philos 1999;24:34–42.

[4] Faden R, Beachamp T. A history and theory of informed consent. New York: Oxford University Press; 1986.

[5] *Canterbury v Spense*, 464 F2d 772, 785 (DC Cir 1972).

[6] Jones JW, McCullough LB. Disclosure of intraoperative events. Surgery 2002;132:531–2.

[7] McKneally MF, Martin DK. An entrustment model of consent for surgical treatment of life-threatening illness: perspective of patients requiring esophagectomy. J Thorac Cardiovasc Surg 2000;120:264–9.

[8] Moseley JB, O'Malley K, Petersen NJ, et al. A controlled trial of arthroscopic surgery for osteoarthritis of the knee. N Engl J Med 2002;347:81–8.

[9] Wear S. Informed consent: patient autonomy and physician beneficence with clinical medicine. Dordrecht: Kluwer Academic Publishers; 1993.

[10] McCullough L, Wilson B, Teasdale NL, et al. Mapping personal, familial, and professional values in long-term care decisions. Gerontologist 1993;33:324–32.

[11] Jones JW, McCullough LB. Refusal of life-saving treatment in the aged. J Vasc Surg 2002;35:1067.

[12] Jones JW, McCullough LB, Richman BW. Management of disagreements between attending and consulting physicians. J Vasc Surg 2003;38:1137–8.

[13] Jones JW, McCullough LB, Richman BW. The surgeon's obligations to the noncompliant patient. J Vasc Surg 2003;38:626–7.

[14] Buchanan A, Brock D. Deciding for others: the ethics of surrogate decision making. New York: Cambridge University Press; 1989.

[15] Areen J. The legal status of consent obtained from families of adult patients to withhold or withdraw treatment. JAMA 1987;258:229–35.

[16] Hare J, Pratt C, Nelson C. Agreement between patients and their self-selected surrogates on difficult medical decisions. Arch Intern Med 1992;152:1049–54.

[17] Committee on Bioethics, American Academy of Pediatrics. Informed consent, parental permission, and assent in pediatric practice. Pediatrics 1995;95:314–7.

[18] Bard S. A discourse upon the duties of a physician. In: Bard S, editor. Two discourses dealing with medical education in early New York. New York: Columbia University Press; 1921.

[19] Jones JW, McCullough LB. Consent for residents to perform surgery. J Vasc Surg 2002;36: 655–6.

[20] Sade RM. Publication of unethical research studies: the importance of informed consent. Ann Thorac Surg 2003;75:325–8.

SURGICAL
CLINICS OF
NORTH AMERICA

Surg Clin N Am 87 (2007) 919–936

Withdrawing Life-Sustaining Treatment: Ethical Considerations

Sharon Reynolds, RN, BA, BScN, MHSc[a,b,*],
Andrew B. Cooper, MD, MHSc[c,d],
Martin McKneally, MD, PhD[a]

[a]Joint Centre for Bioethics, University of Toronto, 88 College Street, Toronto,
Ontario M5G 1L4, Canada
[b]Medical-Surgical Intensive Care Unit, Toronto General Hospital, 585 University Avenue,
Toronto, Ontario M5G 2N2, Canada
[c]The Interdisciplinary Division of Critical Care Medicine, University of Toronto,
Toronto, Ontario, Canada
[d]Sunnybrook and Women's College Health Sciences Centre, M3-200, 2075 Bayview Avenue,
Toronto, Ontario M4N 3M5, Canada

Withdrawing life-supporting technology from patients who are irremediably ill is morally troubling for caregivers, patients, and families. Interventions that enable clinicians to delay death create situations in which the dignity and comfort of dying patients may be sacrificed to spare professionals and families from their elemental fear of death. Understanding of the limits of treatment, expertise in palliation of symptoms, skillful communication, and careful orchestration of controllable events can help to manage the withdrawal of life support appropriately.

Case illustration

You have known your patient Sid for a long time; it seems forever. For 6 months, following an esophagectomy for cancer, his course has been marked by severe complications. Necrosis at the gastroesophageal anastomosis led to an enterocutaneous fistula. Ten subsequent operations and multiple consultants have failed to improve his condition. His chest wall drains continuously, and he has lost 42 pounds. During physiotherapy he

This article originally appeared in the Thoracic Surgery Clinics, November 2005.

* Corresponding author. Joint Centre for Bioethics, University of Toronto, 88 College Street, Toronto, Ontario M5G IL4, Canada.

E-mail address: sharon.reynolds@utoronto.ca (S. Reynolds).

despondently told his nurse "I just want to die." Not long after, he developed pneumonia and was transferred back to the ICU for mechanical ventilation. Two days later, you agreed with his wife and son that a do-not-resuscitate order is appropriate. After a trial of therapy on the ventilator for 2 weeks, the family asked you to call a halt to the life support including vasoactive therapy, antibiotics, and mechanical ventilation. Although Sid was not a capable decision-maker at this point, their feeling was that his earlier statements of despair justified their decision on his behalf.

Why is withdrawal of life support so hard to do?

Because technology has become so effective at extending life, it is difficult to determine when it is appropriate to accept that a patient is dying, cease further aggressive treatment, and strengthen palliative support. A host of issues contribute to the difficulty of withdrawing life-sustaining treatments: the distinction between withholding and withdrawing treatment, religious and cultural considerations, the technologic imperative, prognostic uncertainty, variability in practice, and caregiver discomfort with death. This article focuses on the withdrawal of life-sustaining treatment, because this is the more problematic area for health care providers.

Withdrawing versus withholding life support

Despite consensus that there is no ethical or legal distinction between withholding and withdrawing treatment [1–6], caregivers experience a disturbing difference between the two in practice [5,7–9]. The determining factor is the need for human agency in withdrawal. A trusted and responsible member of the care team must take action and disconnect the ventilator or turn off the inotropic medications supporting blood pressure. This action may lead to immediate death. The feeling of responsibility and culpability for the death that follows is almost inescapable despite theoretical distinctions, professional endorsements, and legal precedents. Seymour [8] followed ICU physicians on their daily rounds and observed their end-of-life decision-making processes. Unless the patient was very close to death, physicians were not comfortable withdrawing support even though they had earlier acknowledged a grim prognosis. They believed they were justified in withdrawing treatment only when "it becomes clear that death will occur in spite of any further treatment maneuvers. In this way a causative link between non-treatment and death is avoided."

To withdraw life support is to recognize that the underlying disease process cannot be reversed. The intention is not to kill, although death certainly ensues. The intention is to acknowledge the limits of medicine. The death that follows, even if immediate, indicates the severity of the disease state and uncovers the inability of the patient's body to survive. Life-support measures mask this reality, and routine interventions that cannot reverse the underlying disease process may confuse families, who often associate ongoing treatment with hope for recovery. Care-related activities that focus on intravenous drips, monitoring lines, and equipment are consoling routines for caregivers even as death becomes inevitable and disease "overmasters the patient." Withdrawal in this setting is a courageous but distressing act of kindness.

Religious and cultural considerations

Religious views may influence decisions to withdraw life-sustaining treatments. It is important to determine the religious beliefs held by the patient or family. One needs to know what their beliefs mean in the context of the present situation. If they are uncertain, yet they wish to adhere to the tenets of their chosen religion, they may need to consult a religious representative within that tradition. Belonging to a specific faith community does not necessarily mean that the patient subscribes to all or any of the tenets of that faith. Most religious outlooks on life share a belief in the sanctity of human life, as a gift from God. Sanctity of life may mean different things to different people. Life has supreme value, for example, in Orthodox Jewish tradition. In this view, withdrawal of supportive therapies is not permissible unless the patient's death, defined by cessation of the heartbeat, is imminent [10–12]. Life-sustaining treatments that are available should be sought [13,14]. Quality-of-life arguments supporting withdrawal of care have no meaning in this context, because the quality of one's life does not define the value of a human being. Within this perspective tube feeding a patient in a persistent vegetative state is morally obligatory care unless the patient is deemed terminally ill (terminal illness in Jewish law is understood as a life expectancy of 3 months [14]) and considered to be suffering. Brain death, as a definition of the termination of life, is not universally accepted [15]. It is very difficult for some people to be told that their loved one is dead yet he or she has a pulse and a blood pressure [16,17].

Religious views are thought to underlie the observation that physicians from Greece, Italy, and Portugal are less inclined to withdraw life-sustaining treatments. "Physicians with a Catholic background were less likely to withhold and withdraw therapy than their Protestant or agnostic counterparts" [18].

Attitudes among laypersons toward life-sustaining interventions were surveyed with scenario questionnaires. Korean Americans believe that life support should always be considered even though this is not what they would choose for themselves. African Americans believe that life-sustaining interventions could be forgone, yet they themselves want such interventions. Within the Chinese culture it is considered rude and courting bad luck to disclose a fatal diagnosis to a patient, obviating direct discussion of withdrawal [19]. Health care providers can initiate conversation that reveals these personal belief systems to guide clinicians in how to speak to patients and what treatments to provide.

Technology: a moral obligation

Significant advances in medical technology and the treatment of disease have changed the goal of medicine from treating what can be treated and respecting what cannot be treated to one of combating death [20]. Technology can be seductive. It can create the illusion of providing certainty and reducing ambiguity. "Like the broom in The Sorcerer's Apprentice, technologies come to have a life of their own..." [21], transforming and dehumanizing the dying process.

The technical components of clinical practice and the myriad interventions possible in a given patient's care represent what can be done to hold death at bay. The question of what ought to be done is grounded in value systems. Disagreements about the right thing to do that arise in this meeting place between value systems and technology can often be reconciled through ethics consultation.

The availability of technology may create a sense of moral obligation to use it based on a belief that to treat is to care. In contrast, clinicians feel responsible, even culpable, if they choose to use technology and then withdraw it. This reasoning leads one to value technology more "than competent compassionate care at the end of life..." [22]. In some ways the intuitive and clinically rooted notions of what is happening to the body of a patient are not trusted. Clinicians feel morally obligated to continue technologic support despite unlikely survival. "Whereas nature once decided who would live or die, our technological capacities have come to play that role" [20] in resource-rich countries. Where there are fewer technologic resources, end-of-life decisions are made with less certainty and conflict.

Prognostic uncertainty

Uncertainty contributes to the dominance of technology in medicine [21]. Decisions to withdraw therapy are based on predictions of future events, deduced from general rules applied to an individual who may not fit that generalization precisely. Because a decision to withdraw treatment becomes irreversible when death occurs, prognostic uncertainty is less tolerable than it is in other domains of medical practice. Prognostic tools, such as Apache II to predict survival probability, do not "provide sufficient power to discriminate accurately between non-survivors and survivors" [23]. When Apache II scores were used with ICU patients on day 1 of admission, "the false positive prediction rate was 7.6% (9 of 118)." A positive prediction rate of 92.4%, although high, does not eliminate the risk of error. In another investigation of predictors of death in critical care units, treatment was withdrawn from 166 patients who were predicted by physicians to die. Six (3.6%) patients in this group eventually left hospital [24]. When compared with validated outcome prediction rules, the physician's own prediction of an adverse prognostic or cognitive function outcome, rather than a score, was the strongest predictor of death. The irreducible nature of uncertainty should not prevent accomplishing a right action. Instead it brings a duty to reflect with the family on the low probability of survival and the poor quality and short duration of residual life.

Physicians generally deal with uncertainty by choosing a course that maximizes potential benefit and minimizes the risk of complications or death. "Clinicians help families by acknowledging prognostic uncertainty directly and by building on that uncertainty to expand the discussion beyond an exclusive focus on survival" [25].

Variability in practice

In addition to uncertainty about outcomes, variabilities in the practice of withdrawing life support are "caused by the idiosyncratic values, beliefs and habits of individual physicians" [8]. Even when physicians use the best evidence available, "their own ethical, social, moral, and religious values influence their medical decision making" [26]. Most Pennsylvania physicians chose to withdraw therapy so that death occurs in subsequent days rather than immediately. Diagnostic uncertainty was a potent factor in the decision. When uncertainty was not a concern, most physicians chose death in 15 minutes over death in 4 hours. Other important factors influencing decision making in this study were defensive motivation (physicians were less likely to withdraw a treatment supporting an organ system that had failed because of iatrogenic complications) and duration of prior therapy. Physicians were less likely to withdraw therapies that had been in place for a long time [27]. Underlining the idiosyncratic and seemingly arbitrary decision-making process regarding withdrawal, a survey of Canadian critical care physicians found that, "in only one of 12 scenarios did more than 50% of the respondents make the same treatment choice" [26].

Legal perspectives

Legal recourse is a last resort when differences of opinion about withdrawing life-sustaining treatment cannot be resolved by other means. The courts tend to support the autonomous rights of patients or their surrogates to make decisions consistent with the value systems of the patients.

In the case of Nancy B., the court faced a conflict when asked to honor the autonomous decision-making rights of a competent patient asking to be disconnected from a ventilator that was sustaining her life. The right to refuse life-sustaining treatment is embodied in the legal doctrine of informed consent [4]. Nancy B. was a 25-year-old woman who had suffered from Guillain-Barré disease for 2.5 years. The conflict in this case existed between a patient's autonomous right to refuse life-sustaining treatments and Section 14 of the Criminal Code, which states that no person may consent to an act that results in their death. The Criminal Code equated withdrawal with euthanasia. This prohibits physicians from ever withdrawing treatment. Mr. Justice Dufour of the Quebec Superior Court needed to find a way to reconcile this conflict. He did so not by interpreting Nancy B.'s request as a request for physician-assisted suicide "but, rather, as an attempt merely to allow a disease to take its natural course" [28]. This case establishes in law that it is the underlying disease that causes the death, not the physician who withdraws unwanted life-supporting treatment.

The case of Helga Wanglie provided further evidence of court support for the decision-making rights of the patient with her husband acting as her surrogate. Helga Wanglie was an 87-year-old woman who had developed pneumonia and respiratory failure following hip replacement surgery. Five months later she suffered a cardiac arrest and never regained consciousness. In June 1990, 1 month after her arrest, physicians sought court permission to discontinue her ventilatory support because Helga could not be weaned from the ventilator and was believed to be in a persistent vegetative state. Her husband argued that physicians are not God and "Only He who gave life has the right to take life." The court supported Mr. Wanglie as best able to represent his wife's interests. Helga died 7 days after the court decision [29]. Current practice supports respecting value systems and beliefs that honor sanctity of life. As resource constraints increase, these issues will be debated publicly.

Physicians made a unilateral decision to place a do-not-resuscitate order on the chart of 72-year-old Catherine Gilgunn, against the wishes of her daughter. The patient's medical history included diabetes, heart disease, Parkinson's disease, and cerebrovascular disease. Refractory seizures had rendered her irreversibly comatose. Hospital lawyers supported the decision of the physician to instate a do-not-resuscitate order despite disagreement from the patient's daughter. The decision was believed to be in the "patient's best interests." When her daughter took legal action against her mother's physicians and the hospital, the Superior Court of Massachusetts supported the medical team. The physicians argued that their decision to withhold nonbeneficial treatment was "consistent with professional standards" [30]. Despite this finding by the court, unilateral decision making is not recommended [31,32], especially in withdrawal of life support.

Recently, Laura Hawryluck, an intensive care physician, asked permission of the court to remove the daughters of her patient as decision makers for their irreversibly demented mother who has required repeated admissions to the ICU for ventilatory support during recurrent bouts of pneumonia. Given the frequent dependence on ICU intervention and the inability to reverse the underlying disease process, Dr. Hawryluck asked for permission to focus on palliative support on a hospital ward instead of ICU care. The court ruled against Dr. Hawryluck, supporting the request of the family for ICU care consistent with their mother's religious views (a link to the Hawryluck case is http://www.canlii.org/on/cas/onsc/2004/2004onsc10339.html).

Can physicians refuse to provide care that is clearly prolonging death and not of benefit? Perhaps "terminally ill patients do not have the right to demand any and all treatments" [33]. There are guidelines provided by the American Thoracic Society and the Society of Critical Care Medicine regarding the withdrawal of treatment in situations considered futile. A physician is not morally obligated to initiate or continue a treatment considered not to be of benefit to a patient or to yield a quality of life not acceptable to the patient. It is suggested that consent of the patient or surrogate decision maker is not required [34–36]. Proceeding without consent remains legally problematic.

Downie [32] argues that there is "an urgent need for lawmakers to clarify when doctors have the right to withhold and withdraw their services." Health care providers are currently stuck in a gray zone on these issues.

The withdrawal process: how to do it

Because withdrawal of life support typically happens when patients have become incapable of communicating directly with clinicians, the process usually involves substitute decision making with the patient's family [25]. Estimates of the proportion of patients involved in decision making under these circumstances vary in the literature from 6% to 35% [37,38]. Few critically ill patients arrive in the ICU with explicit advance directives [39] and, where present, the language of an advanced care directive may lack power to address the particulars of the patient's circumstances. Even if an advance directive exists, the personal values it reflects may change in altered circumstances. Preferences in the new situation cannot be assumed to be identical to those in an advance directive. Despite a reasonable likelihood of success for resuscitative therapy, patients modify their choices in light of the accompanying disability. As the burden of disability increases, fewer patients choose to be resuscitated [40]. Empirical data underlie the importance of meticulous informed consent for high-risk surgical procedures. Beyond the usual discussion of postoperative complications, the possibility of a prolonged ICU stay with its attendant burdens of suffering [41] should be discussed, including an exploration of the patient's preferences should survival with severe disability be the outcome. A well-documented preoperative discussion of patient preferences when considering withdrawal of life support in the context of anticipated degrees of disability can inform action in the patient's best interest. One of us (MM) has engaged in this practice for many years. Most patients are grateful for the opportunity to discuss this possibility. A small number are unable to address it, because they are already overwhelmed by thinking about their illness and its treatment.

Although there are rare circumstances in which it may be possible to awaken critically ill patients to discuss treatment options, this is usually not practical. Sepsis itself may impair capacity and severe hypoxemia that accompanies respiratory failure in critical illness makes reversal of sedative medication effects problematic, mainly because of the difficulty in maintaining patient ventilator synchrony. Hepatic and renal dysfunction, altered volumes of distribution, and reduced protein binding may delay clearance of centrally acting drugs. The obligation to involve patients in their care decisions, based on the principle of respect for persons, must be balanced against the suffering that removal of sedation and analgesia may cause during a terminal critical illness [42].

Communication with families of critically ill patients about withdrawal of life support is not easy. A useful reflective taxonomy is to consider physician, environmental, and family factors contributing to inadequate communication. There is a growing literature on the inadequacy of physician communication in this setting. When family conferences are studied, physicians dominate the discussion. In some instances, up to 70% of the content is uttered by the physician. There are frequent physician-induced turns of conversation [43]. Physicians miss opportunities in about one third of family conferences to be empathic, to listen to family concerns, and to address key principles of palliative care [44].

Ideally, responsible staff physicians should conduct family conferences in the presence of house staff and nurses. Families of patients find information conveyed by junior staff less satisfactory and less understandable compared with discussions held with attending physicians. They are likely to require additional communication if the initial contact is by a junior doctor [45]. Compared with satisfaction with nurse communication, family satisfaction with physician communication is modest but improves as the number of physician visits increases [46]. "The virtue of being present" is a theme expressed throughout the literature on withdrawal of life support in the ICU and elsewhere in palliative care medicine. Families of critically ill patients are often overwhelmed by exposure to the information-dense environment of the ICU and their concern for a loved one. The prevalence of anxiety and depression is high, reaching nearly 70% when both symptoms are considered together [47]. Emotional distress may interfere with capacity of family members to act as substitute decision makers. Families are more likely to experience effective communication when it is conducted in a private conference room than when sensitive discussions are conducted in public places like hallways. The bedside in the ICU is unsuitable; there is a high likelihood of interruptions and distractions [48] and paroxysmal noise levels sometimes exceeding 70 dB [49], the equivalent of busy street corners.

Communication with distressed families to discuss limits of treatment requires specialized skills and attitudes on the part of the physician. Although many of these skills are in the domain of social workers, hospital chaplains, or bioethicists, the attending surgeon or physician is medically and legally responsible and accountable for decisions about treatment.

Essential skills include the ability to establish trust, to appreciate affective moments and show empathy, and to communicate medical facts in nontechnical language. Ideally, the surgeon engages family decision makers in a dialog about reasonable treatment options, reflective of the goals and health-related values of the patient; the deliberative physician patient relationship is most appropriate when there is adequate time and commitment [50]. The importance of relationship as a vehicle for creating trust means that arriving at a shared plan takes time and commitment to ongoing dialog. The empathic response to expressions of emotion is to state simply that one has noticed the emotion and to express acceptance and appreciation that it is appropriate [51]. During family conferences, silence is often more valuable than words. When disagreements emerge among family members or between the health care team and the family in a conference, deliberately allowing silence to develop is an excellent way to refocus the discussion. Silence in the context of empathic communication gives the patient's family the experience of being understood [52]. Silence enlightens and enlivens ethical reflection.

Dealing with requests for euthanasia

Four hours after extubation, the bedside nurse calls you to express her concern that Sid is struggling for air. She tells you that in 11 years of ICU nursing she has never witnessed so much suffering in a dying patient. "He seems to be indestructible. I cannot imagine what it will take to end his suffering, unless it's something like KCL." The family at the bedside looks up at you despairingly.

Outside critical care settings, surveys in the United States, Britain, and Australia reveal that about one quarter of physicians and nurses are approached by patients or families at some time with requests for active euthanasia or physician-assisted death. Of these respondents, a small proportion accommodates the requests. Within critical care units, one survey of a random sample of 1600 nurses subscribing to the journal *Nursing* (readership 500,000) revealed that 17% had received such requests. Of those who received requests, 16% accommodated them, sometimes by pretending to provide life-sustaining treatment while omitting it. The investigators estimated that about 7% of nurses involved in these activities initiated them without the knowledge of decision makers, claiming tacit consent [53]. Without clear guidance on quality end-of-life care, idiosyncratic solutions are the norm.

A combination of factors, such as nonacceptance of death, the virtuous desire to relieve suffering, and lack of confidence in the training and ability of physicians to control symptoms at the end of life, lead to the conclusion that the only solution seems to be active euthanasia. A study of 36 patients followed by a university palliative care service revealed only about two thirds of patients rated their care as very good or excellent [54]. The same investigators found that priorities for improvement were in domains of symptom control (pain, shortness of breath, thirst, and other symptoms); reducing delays (in care, diagnosis, and transfer home); better access to their physicians and nurses (for information and improved therapeutic alliances); and the addressing of emotional concerns, such as loneliness and fear of abandonment. Quantification of the quality of death is possible and offers insight into what can be done to improve the practice of withdrawal of life support. A systematically developed measurement tool quality of death and dying highlights key patient-identified preferences for end-of-life care [55]. The quality of death in the ICU falls far short of what is valued by dying patients. Palliative care in the ICU differs from care in other settings, because the dying process is more dramatic or linked to medical decision-making, and because the time from initiation of the process to death is usually shorter. There are special problems in the assessment of pain and suffering in ICU patients: communication problems, severity of illness, decreased levels of consciousness, and difficulty interpreting the usual clinical signs of distress [56].

The focus in the practice of withdrawal of life support should be on those items that can be changed; symptom control (pain and dyspnea); preparation for death (supporting the family and offering spiritual care); the conduct of death (inviting family to be present); ending unwanted therapies; and encouraging physical contact as the transition occurs. Palliative care initiatives can address the shortcomings that bring about requests for active euthanasia and physician assisted death in critically ill patients.

Symptom control during withdrawal of life support

You return to the bedside, where Sid is gasping for breath. His systolic blood pressure is 50 mm Hg, and despite high doses of midazolam (320 mg) and an increase in the hydromorphone infusion to 500 mg/h he still is apparently in severe distress.

Physicians attempting to relieve symptoms in dying patients tread a difficult path; if not enough medication is given, there is the risk of inadequate symptom control. If too much is given, there is the risk of being accused of practicing active euthanasia or physician-assisted death. The dosages mentioned previously were administered to a dying patient in Canada. Responding to the distress of the patient, his family, and the bedside nurse, a physician decided to hasten death with medication devoid of analgesic or anxiolytic effect: potassium chloride. In the testimony of expert witnesses during an inquiry to determine whether the physician would be committed to stand trial for first-degree murder, drug dosages were a focus of testimony. Two days before the patient's death, procedural pain during an incision and drainage had been relieved with only fractions of the previously mentioned amounts: 5 mg of hydromorphone and 2 mg of midazolam.

The patient's body was exhumed in the investigation, but a toxicology report found only "traces of dilaudid and morphine in the liver." A critical care physician who testified pointed out that the apparent ineffectiveness of such large doses of medication should have prompted an investigation of the effectiveness of the intravenous access used to administer medications for symptom control [57]. The first practice point in symptom control during withdraw of life support is to review the medication history, determining the treatments in use and the patient's responses both at rest and during stimulation. This guides the practitioner toward an appropriate starting point for symptom control. Next, inspection of the intravenous access is important. In edematous patients it may be difficult to determine whether existing peripheral intravenous lines are intravascular or interstitially placed. If there is doubt, it is prudent to replace them or to ensure they are functioning appropriately before relying on them in withdrawing life support. Injecting a bolus of a marker, such as a rapidly cleared vasoactive drug (eg, phenylephrine, 100 µg, if not contraindicated), may help to clarify the adequacy of existing catheters without the delay associated with acquiring a drug level. If this step is necessary, perhaps because of excessive difficulty or risk associated with replacement of existing intravenous access, it is important explicitly to declare the intention associated with the injection of the marker dose in the orders and the patient care record. When writing orders for symptom control it is important to specify indications for all comfort medications to avoid the potential for accusations of assisted euthanasia or physician-assisted death (eg, by writing "for pain and dyspnea" after the opioid and "for anxiety" after the benzodiazepine dosages).

Guidelines on the use of medication in these settings are helpful to maintain practice within the standards of the profession. Table 1 summarizes key points of the statement on end-of-life care of the Society of Critical Care Medicine, and of a Delphi study systematically evaluating the consensus of Canadian Intensive Care specialists, and provincial coroners [56]. The Society of Critical Care Medicine recommendations present a useful taxonomy for commonly encountered scenarios in withdrawal of ventilatory support [58]. It classifies the needs of patients according to neurologic function and the likelihood of dyspnea. There are three possibilities, and the approach to symptom control should be adapted accordingly (Table 2).

Symptom control in paralyzed patients

Many of the signs of pain and suffering in dying patients are masked by neuromuscular paralysis. Canadian and American expert opinion concurs that the use of neuromuscular blockade to mask the signs of death or to initiate withdraw of life support while neuromuscular blockade is still present is unethical [56,58,59]. Even under optimal conditions it is hard to monitor and correctly interpret bedside tests of neuromuscular function. Pre-emptive treatment of pain and suffering is appropriate if patients have been receiving

Table 1
Management of pain and suffering

Relief of pain and suffering	Nonpharmacologic means	Pharmacologic means
Relief of pain and suffering	Ensure presence of friends, family, pastoral care	Analgesics, sedatives, adjuncts
	Change technologic environment	Treat pain, suffering or both with appropriate agents
Initial dosages	Individualize Therapy ∝	See below for summary of pharmacology
	Narcotic exposure, age, prior alcohol, drug use	
	Organ dysfunction	
	Level of consciousness	
	Level of psychologic support	
	Wishes for sedation during death	
Titration of sedatives and analgesics	Increase doses in response to signs	Limitations of clinical indicators
	Doses may exceed preconceived notions	Imprecise
	Patient's request	Supplement with VAS pain, RASS scale
	Tachycardia, hypertension, sweating	
	Facial grimacing, tears, vocalization with movement	
	Restlessness	
Maximum doses	Maximum doses do not exist[a]	The intent of the treating physician distinguishes palliative care from AE, PAD
	If specified, some patients may suffer with inadequate symptom control	
Pre-emptive or responsive therapy?	Clear documentation of intention is required	Pre-emptive dosing in anticipation of pain or suffering is good palliative care, not AE

Abbreviations: AE, active euthanasia; PAD, physician assisted death; RASS, Richmond agitation-sedation scale; VAS, visual analogue scale.

[a] In one case series of terminal weaning of chronic ventilator-dependent patients, morphine doses given during withdraw of life support ranged from 2–50 mg and benzodiazepine doses ranged from 8–675 mg.

neuromuscular blockade and continue to manifest paralysis despite discontinuation of drug infusions.

Conflict resolution and family demands for inappropriate treatment

It is normal for conflicts to occur at the end of life. Accepting this allows the team to look at conflict from a broader perspective. Death of the person becomes a prominent part of illness narratives before death of the physical body [60]. The stages of the grieving process, which in premodern times occurred after death, are displaced by life support to the period before death. Grief can be expressed through conflict in discussions about the futility of treatment as the family encounters and struggles with the impending loss of their beloved.

Table 2
Anticipation and treatment of discomfort in withdrawal of life support

Neurologic function	Likelihood of distress	Technique
Brain death	None; possibility of lazarus reflexes	Extubation; preparation of family
Comatose patients	Uncertain	Extubation or rapid ↓ support; ± sedation
Conscious patients	High	Gradual ↓ support; titrate sedation

Families have the opportunity to discuss care with a diversity of teams in the ICU. The composition and structure of these teams is complex and their membership frequently changes. Differences in sensitivity to the needs of families may bring about conflict. Continuity and consistency in communication is often difficult to maintain. Physicians in the ICU do not communicate well with each other. They miss opportunities for direct communication and use intermediaries, such as trainees or the chart, for important messages. Leaving a consulting service "out of the loop" with regard to the content of important family conferences can result in the communication of inconsistent messages to families. Families struggle with difficult personal, emotional, or religious aspects, whereas teams encounter challenges in regard to their authority in the decision-making process. Shared medical responsibility among several teams leads to problems in giving clear guidance to families. Families, who may value intensive care as an expression of devotion to the person or as part of religious duty, are confused and offended when team members seem to undervalue their technologic interventions based on medical effectiveness.

A series of penetrating questions that explore family, physician, and institutional or social influences contributing to the conflict is discussed in a scheme for the differential diagnosis of conflicts as outlined in Box 1 [61]. This scheme for differential diagnosis presents a useful framework for the exploration of the family's experience of illness and opens the door to the creation of a therapeutic narrative in which their experience is acknowledged and validated. It also gives guidelines for the physician, highlighting areas in which support may be needed.

Summary

In the community of caregivers, there is a general consensus that some heroic measures are not obligatory in certain circumstances that are defined by professional norms. For example, cardiopulmonary resuscitation in terminal cancer patients is not endorsed because of its violation of the dignity of the irremediably ill, and its unproductive cost to society. Moving back from this extreme, the availability and effectiveness of life-prolonging treatments, such as ventilators, dialysis, and implantable mechanical hearts, moves into a domain where the boundary limit of the obligation to preserve

Box 1. Accepting conflict and creating dialogue

Ask the family:
What do you understand about what is going on?
Why have you decided to _____?
What are you hoping we can accomplish/achieve?
What do you think _____ would want us to accomplish for him/
     her?
What else would he/she want us to accomplish?
Which, of these, are the most important?
In what situations, if any, could you imagine _____ not wanting to
     continue to live?
Are your questions getting answered? Do you have concerns
     about the care you/your loved one is getting?
Are there disagreements among family members?

Ask yourself:
What do I think are this patient's chances of surviving
     to discharge recovering function?
What have I told the patient/family are his/her chances
     of surviving to discharge/recovering function?
How sure am I about his/her prognosis? On what is it based?
What do I know about what this patient wants or would have
     wanted? How do I know? How sure am I?
Is this patient competent to make his/her own decisions? How do
     I know? How sure am I? Could it be fluctuating or reversible
     incompetence?
Did I/we contribute to a bad outcome in any way (eg, missed
     diagnosis, delayed treatment)?
How do I feel about discussing this patient's death with him/her
     (his/her family)?
Who is this patient's "family doctor"? Clergy of choice? Primary
     nurse? Social worker?
Do I feel I have enough time to talk to the patient/family about
     prognosis, options, and goals?
What words or phrases have I (for others) used that might be
     contributing to the conflict (eg, "stopping treatment," "comfort
     measures only," "hopeless," "certain")?
What aspectist of this patient's life do I feel justify withholding
     or withdrawing life-sustaining treatment?
Does the family trust us? If not, why not?

Ask about social/organizational influences:
Are there financial pressures on the family?
Are there financial pressures on the hospital?

Are there financial pressures on the medical team?
Are families allowed to see what the patient's day is like?
Are there any concerns about malpractice or legality?
Are there cultural or religious differences among the patient/
family/physicians/hospital?

From Goold SD, Williams B, Arnold RM. Conflicts regarding decisions to limit
treatment: a differential diagnosis. JAMA 2000;283:909–14; with permission.

life is less clearly defined. When the continuing intervention of caregivers is
essential to the prolongation of life, but the outcome and quality of residual
life has deteriorated far below everyone's expectations when the treatment
was initiated, caregivers are morally troubled as their treatments prolong
the process of dying.

Uncertainty or disputation about the prognosis raises the voltage of the
fear and potential remorse that is a normal condition of care and support at
the end of life. Unilateral decisions and overruling of objections should be
avoided when possible, and reinforced by legal or ethical authorities when
necessary. An ethics consultant, especially one skilled and experienced in
management of end-of-life issues, can be a helpful negotiator and guide.

The transition to palliative support should include the discontinuation of
all unnecessary monitoring devices and tubes. Monitors should be turned off
allowing families to direct their attention to the patient. Removing the monitor relieves family members from painful suspense and confusion. Removing the endotracheal tube sometimes allows conscious patients to talk to
their loved ones, ending a silence forced on them by their treatment. If
interventions are seen as masking the natural dying process, removing
them should not be troubling. Their absence gives moral clarity to the elemental moments of closure at the end of life, no longer masked by futile
contrivance.

Withdrawal of life-sustaining treatment is a process that "merits the same
meticulous preparation and expectation of quality that clinicians provide
when they perform other procedures to initiate life support" [6]. Families
and patients should never feel abandoned during this process and attention
should be devoted to communicating that care is not being withdrawn. The
family needs to be prepared for what the dying process may look like.
Assure them that all energy is now being directed toward the comfort of
the patient including sedation as required if signs of suffering are observed.

Easing death, like easing birth, can be one of the most fulfilling contributions one can make to reduce the suffering and enrich the lives of patients
and their families. Neglecting this part of the duty to provide appropriate
care brings moral anguish to all participants in the peculiar circumstances
that have come to surround death in the ICUs of developed countries.

It is helpful to accept the inevitable reality that death is, in Shakespeare's words, a "necessary end" to all mortal life, and to recognize that defying death with technology can sometimes become an unnatural and degrading activity, however well motivated. The withdrawal of life-sustaining treatment, when conducted expertly, is a shared human experience that can be gratifying, although difficult for all concerned.

References

[1] Beauchamp TL, Childress JF. Principles of biomedical ethics. 5th edition. New York: Oxford University Press; 2001.

[2] Rieth KA. How do we withhold or withdraw life-sustaining therapy? Nurs Manage 1999;30: 20–5.

[3] Prien T, Van Aken H. Ethical dilemmas in intensive care: can the problem be solved? Curr Opin Anaesthesiol 1999;12:203–6.

[4] Gostin LO. Deciding life and death in the courtroom: from Quinlan to Cruzan, Glucksberg, and Vacco. A brief history and analysis of constitutional protection of the 'right to die'. JAMA 1997;278:1523–8.

[5] Vincent J. Cultural differences in end-of-life care. Crit Care Med 2001;29:N52–5.

[6] Rubenfeld GD, Crawford SW. Principles and practice of withdrawing life-sustaining treatment in the ICU. In: Curtis RJ, Rubenfeld GD, editors. Managing death in the ICU the transition from cure to comfort. New York: Oxford University Press; 2001. p. 127–47.

[7] Gordon M. Whose life is it and who decides? A dilemma in long-term care. Annals of Long Term Care 2004;9:1524.

[8] Seymour JE. Negotiating natural death in intensive care. Soc Sci Med 2000;51:1241–52.

[9] Melltorp G, Nilstun T. The difference between withholding and withdrawing life-sustaining treatment. Intensive Care Med 1997;23:1264–7.

[10] Rosner F. Jewish medical ethics. J Clin Ethics 1995;6:202–17.

[11] Morrison MF, Demichele SG. How culture and religion affect attitudes toward medical futility. In: Zucker MB, Zucker HD, editors. Medical futility and the evaluation of life-sustaining interventions. New York: Cambridge University Press; 1997. p. 71–82.

[12] Clarfield AM, Gordon M, Markwell H, et al. Ethical issues in end-of-life geriatric care: the approach of three monotheistic religions: Judaism, Catholicism, and Islam. Journal of American Geriatrics Society 2003;51:1149–54.

[13] Weijer C. CPR for patient's in a PVS: futile or acceptable? Can Med Assoc J 1998;158:491–3.

[14] Kunin J. Withholding artificial feeding from the severely demented: merciful or immoral? contrasts between secular and Jewish perspectives. J Med Ethics 2003;29:208–12.

[15] Truog RD, Fackler JC. It is reasonable to reject the diagnosis of brain death. J Clin Ethics 1992;3:80–1.

[16] Kirkland LL. Brain death and the termination of life support: case and analysis. J Clin Ethics 1992;3:78.

[17] Freer JP. Brain death and the termination of life support: case and analysis. J Clin Ethics 1992;3:78.

[18] Vincent J. Forgoing life support in western European intensive care units: the results of an ethical questionnaire. Crit Care Med 1999;27:1626–33.

[19] Levin PD, Sprung CL. Cultural differences at the end of life. Crit Care Med 2003;31:S354–7.

[20] Callahan D. The troubled dream of life: in search of a peaceful death. Washington: Georgetown University Press; 2000.

[21] Cassell EJ. The sorcerer's broom: medicine's rampant technology. Hastings Cent Rep 1993; 23:32–9.

[22] Nelson JE, Danis M. End-of-life care in the intensive care unit: where are we now? Crit Care Med 2001;29(2 Suppl):N2–9.

[23] Wong DT, Gomez M, Mcguire GP, et al. Utilization of intensive care unit days in a Canadian medical-surgical intensive care unit. Crit Care Med 1999;27:1319–24.

[24] Cook D, Rocker G, Marshall J, et al. Withdrawal of mechanical ventilation in anticipation of death in the intensive care unit. N Engl J Med 2003;349:1123–32.

[25] Prendergast TJ, Puntillo KA. Withdrawal of life support: intensive caring at the end of life. JAMA 2002;288:2732–40.

[26] Cook DJ, Guyatt GH, Jaeschke R, et al. Determinants in Canadian health care workers of the decision to withdraw life support from the critically ill. Canadian Critical Care Trials Group. JAMA 1995;273:703–8.

[27] Christakis NA, Asch DA. Biases in how physicians choose to withdraw life support. Lancet 1993;342:642–7.

[28] Fish A, Singer PA, Nancy B. The criminal code and decisions to forgo life-sustaining treatment. Can Med Assoc J 1992;147:637–42.

[29] Lo B. Resolving ethical dilemmas: a guide for clinicians. Baltimore: Williams & Wilkins; 1995.

[30] Luce JM, Alpers A. Legal aspects of withholding and withdrawing life support from critically ill patients in the United States and providing palliative care to them. Am J Respir Care Med 2000;162:2029–32.

[31] Luce JM, Alpers A. End-of-life care: what do the American courts say? Crit Care Med 2001; 29:N40–5.

[32] Downie J. Unilateral withholding and withdrawal of life-sustaining treatment: a violation of dignity under the law in Canada. J Palliat Care 2004;20:143–9.

[33] Duffy A, Tam P. Patients, doctors in ethical grey zone. The Ottawa Citizen. April 28, 2005.

[34] American Thoracic Society. Withholding and with drawing life-sustaining therapy. Am Rev Respir Dis 1991;144:726–31.

[35] Task Force on Ethics of the Society of Critical Care Medicine. Consensus report on the ethics of foregoing life-sustaining treatments in the critically ill. Crit Care Med 1990;18: 1435–9.

[36] American Medical Association. E-2.037 Medical futility in end-of-life care. www.ama-assn. org/ama/pub/category/8390.html. Accessed July 25, 2005.

[37] Nolin T, Andersson R. Withdrawal of medical treatment in the ICU: a cohort study of 318 cases during 1994–2000. Acta Anaesthesiol Scand 2003;47:501–7.

[38] Faber-Langendoen KA. Multi-institutional study of care given to patients dying in hospitals ethical and practice implications. Arch Intern Med 1996;156:2130–6.

[39] Cook DJ, Guyatt G, Rocker G, et al. Cardiopulmonary resuscitation directives on admission to intensive care unit: an international observational study. Lancet 2001;358:1941–5.

[40] Fried TR, Bradley EH, Towle VR, et al. Understanding the treatment preferences of seriously ill patients. N Engl J Med 2002;346:1061–6.

[41] Rotondi AJ, Chelluri L, Sirio C, et al. Patients' recollections of stressful experiences while receiving prolonged mechanical ventilation in an intensive care unit. Crit Care Med 2002; 30:746–52.

[42] Tonelli MR. Waking the dying: must we always attempt to involve critically ill patients in end-of-life decisions? Chest 2005;127:637–42.

[43] Gottschalk LA, Bechtel RJ, Buchman TG, et al. Computerized content analysis of conversational interactions. Comput Inform Nurs 2003;21:249–58.

[44] Curtis JR, Engelberg RA, Wenrich MD, et al. Missed opportunities during family conferences about end-of-life care in the intensive care unit. Am J Respir Crit Care Med 2005; 171:844–9.

[45] Moreau D, Goldgran-Toledano D, Alberti C, et al. Junior versus senior physicians for informing families of intensive care unit patients. Am J Respir Crit Care Med 2004;169:512–7.

[46] Heyland DK, Rocker GM, Dodek PM, et al. Family satisfaction with care in the intensive care unit: results of a multiple center study. Crit Care Med 2002;30:1413–8.

[47] Pochard F, Azoulay E, Chevret S, et al. Symptoms of anxiety and depression in family members of intensive care unit patients: ethical hypothesis regarding decision-making capacity. Crit Care Med 2001;29:1893–7.

[48] Happ MB, Kagan SH. Methodological considerations for grounded theory research in critical care settings. Nurs Res 2001;50:188–92.

[49] Gabor JY, Cooper AB, Crombach SA, et al. Contribution of the intensive care unit environment to sleep disruption in mechanically ventilated patients and healthy subjects. Am J Respir Crit Care Med 2003;167:708–15.

[50] Emanuel EJ, Emanuel LL. Four models of the physician patient relationship. In: Boetzkes E, Waluchow WJ, editors. Readings in health care ethics, vol. 1. 1st edition. Toronto: Broadview Press; 2000. p. 40–9.

[51] Buckman R. How to break bad news: a guide for health care professionals. Baltimore: The Johns Hopkins University Press; 1992.

[52] Coulehan JL, Platt FW, Egener B, et al. "Let me see if I have this right…": words that help build empathy. Ann Intern Med 2001;135:221–7.

[53] Asch DA. The role of critical care nurses in euthanasia and assisted suicide. N Engl J Med 1996;334:1374–9.

[54] Powis J, Etchells E, Martin DK, et al. Can a "good death" be made better? preliminary evaluation of a patient -centered quality improvement strategy for severely ill in-patients. BMC Palliative Care 2004;3:2–9. Available at: http://www.biomedcentral.com/1472-684X/3/2. Accessed May 8, 2005.

[55] Patrick DL, Engelberg RA, Curtis JR. Evaluating the quality of dying and death. J Pain Symptom Manage 2001;22:717–26.

[56] Hawryluck LA, Harvey WRC, Lemieux-Charles L, et al. Consensus guidelines on analgesia and sedation in dying intensive care unit patients. BMC Medical Ethics 2002;3:3–12. Available at: http://www.biomedcentral.com/1472-6939/3/3. Accessed May 8, 2005.

[57] Sneiderman B, Deutscher R. Dr. Nancy Morrison and her dying patient: a case of medical necessity. Health Law J 2002;10:1–30.

[58] Truog RD, Cist AF, Brackett SE, et al. Recommendations for end-of-life care in the intensive care unit: the Ethics Committee of the Society of Critical Care Medicine. Crit Care Med 2001;29:2332–48.

[59] Riker RR, Fraser GL, Rohr WB, et al. Neuromuscular blockade at the end of life. N Engl J Med 2000;342:1921–2.

[60] Johnson N, Cook D, Giacomini M, et al. Towards a "good" death: end-of-life narratives constructed in an intensive care unit. Cult Med Psychiatry 2000;24:275.

[61] Goold SD, Williams B, Arnold RM. Conflicts regarding decisions to limit treatment: a differential diagnosis. JAMA 2000;283:909–14.

ELSEVIER
SAUNDERS

SURGICAL
CLINICS OF
NORTH AMERICA

Surg Clin N Am 87 (2007) 937–948

The Effect of Patients' Noncompliance on Their Surgeons' Obligations

Jay A. Jacobson, MD, FACP

Division of Medical Ethics, Department of Internal Medicine, LDS Hospital and University of Utah School of Medicine, Salt Lake City, UT 84143, USA

I recently had an instructive encounter with the word, "obligation." Senior medical students had met, heard, and interacted with Paul Farmer, the Tanner Lecturer on human values. Dr. Farmer is an internationally respected physician who has dedicated his life and work to treatment of people in the developing world. More students than could be accommodated responded when invited to have lunch with Dr. Farmer. They eagerly queried him about opportunities to work with underserved populations. The next week in the Medical Ethics course, I asked all 104 students if they believed they had any obligation to serve the world's poorest and most vulnerable populations. I was stunned when no one raised a hand. I acknowledged my surprise and asked them to share their reaction to the question. Many of them expressed interest, willingness, desire, and even a plan to do some medical service in the Third World. All of them, however, took issue with the concept of obligation. They were looking forward to their medical independence and freedom from the regimentation of medical school and the constraints of residency. Maybe it was the added awareness of their enormous loans, but "obligation" triggered strong negative reactions. They recognized that they were obliged to complete residencies to practice medicine, but they did not recognize a universal obligation to serve any particular patient or patient population. They resented the idea that others expected or asserted such a duty.

These soon-to-be physicians were young and inexperienced. They had not yet sworn any oaths, received their licenses, or signed any contracts. Nevertheless, their reactions and comments made me realize that I may have made some assumptions about physicians' obligations to patients that were not widely shared and perhaps not well supported. They reminded me that physicians value their freedom, autonomy, and authority, and do

---

This article originally appeared in the Thoracic Surgery Clinics, November 2005.
E-mail address: jay.jacobson@intermountainmail.org

0039-6109/07/$ - see front matter © 2007 Elsevier Inc. All rights reserved.
doi:10.1016/j.suc.2007.07.014
surgical.theclinics.com

not welcome the idea of being told what to do or being obliged to do it. The students also reminded me that people prefer and enjoy work they want to do more than work they have to do.

Few prefer or enjoy working with "noncompliant" patients, but this article explores whether clinicians, surgeons in particular, are obliged to take care of them. The sources for professional and personal obligations to patients are considered; there are some obligations, but they are specific and contextual. Also examined are what actions exempt surgeons from these obligations and whether noncompliance per se always or sometimes constitutes such an exemption. Because there is an obligation to treat at least some noncompliant patients, ways to identify those patients and strategies to make working with them more effective and less onerous are suggested.

What are surgeons' professional and personal obligations to patients?

Many look to the Hippocratic Oath as a statement of medicine's principles and priorities [1]. It might clarify professional obligations. It pledges that clinicians will act for the benefit of the patient, but it does not explain how someone gets to be the patient. Once someone becomes the patient, the oath obliges one to respect his or her confidence and not reveal embarrassing information. The oath obliges one not to prescribe a deadly drug or to participate in birth control. It is silent about whether noncompliance relieves one of any obligation. The oath may not even be relevant or applicable to surgeons because it was intended for other kinds of physicians, as reflected in the statement: "I will not use the knife, not even on sufferers from stone, but will withdraw in favor of such men as are engaged in this work" [1]. The oath, ostensibly written in the fourth century BC and probably by someone other than Hippocrates, seems more than a bit dated now and does not reflect changes in medical knowledge, technology, ethics, and law. It would not be regarded as binding unless one swore to it and even then there is no real mechanism for monitoring adherence or sanctions based on a breach of this promise.

Most physicians actually take quite a different oath when they complete medical school. Today, the "Oath of Lasagna" is one of several oaths that have been offered to replace the original Hippocratic Oath while preserving its spirit [2]. Other alternatives include the Oath of Maimonides, attributed to the twelfth-century Jewish physician Moses Maimonides [3], and the Declaration of Geneva [4], composed by the World Medical Association in 1948. The latter is, in part, reactive and responsive to the terrible, involuntary medical experiments conducted by German physicians in World War II. The trend among many medical schools is to have each graduating class hammer out an oath of its own that reflects the professional ideals of its members [5]. Although these newer oaths add new obligations, such as securing voluntary, informed consent for research, they make no mention of an obligation to treat all patients. They do not mention noncompliance.

Interestingly, the earliest American Medical Association's (AMA) Code of Ethics in 1847 included what could be regarded as a code of expected behavior for patients [6]. "The obedience of a patient to the prescriptions of his physician should be prompt and implicit. He should never permit his own crude opinions as to their fitness, to influence his attention to them...This remark is equally applicable to diet, drink, and exercise." It urged patients to be compliant with medical instructions. That code also omitted any generic obligation to care for all or a particular class of patients, but it did mention obligations to patients in one's practice. It did not indicate whether patient noncompliance could excuse doctors from these obligations.

The current AMA Code of Ethics reflects the larger changes in American society that have diminished the unquestioned authority of leaders and professionals and elevated the autonomy and rights of individuals and classes of persons, including patients [7]. The long tradition of medical paternalism, doctor knows best, and following doctor's "orders" is no longer widely accepted by the American public or supported by laws related to patient decision making. The AMA Code now has a brief section that includes patient responsibilities. Its language reflects an incomplete transition between an earlier era of doctor-directed care and a currently envisioned negotiated partnership between doctor and patient.

> It has long been recognized that successful medical care requires an ongoing collaborative effort between patients and physicians. Physician and patient are bound in a partnership that requires both individuals to take an active role in the healing process. Such a partnership does not imply that both partners have identical responsibilities or equal power. While physicians have the responsibility to provide health care services to patients to the best of their ability, patients have the responsibility to communicate openly, to participate in decisions about the diagnostic and treatment recommendations, and to comply with the agreed-upon treatment program. Like patients' rights, patients' responsibilities are derived from the principle of autonomy. The principle of patient autonomy holds that an individual's physical, emotional, and psychological integrity should be respected and upheld. This principle also recognizes the human capacity to self-govern and choose a course of action from among different alternative options. Autonomous, competent patients assert some control over the decisions which direct their health care.
>
> ...Once patients and physicians agree upon the goals of therapy and a treatment plan, patients have a responsibility to cooperate with that treatment plan and to keep their agreed-upon appointments. Compliance with physician instructions is often essential to public and individual safety. Patients also have a responsibility to disclose whether previously agreed upon treatments are being followed and to indicate when they would like to reconsider the treatment plan.

Although not stating a universal professional obligation to care for all patients who request it, the current Code, which begins with nine principles, states in number 6: "A physician shall, in the provision of appropriate patient care, except in emergencies, be free to choose whom to serve, with whom to associate, and the environment in which to provide medical care" [8]. This suggests that there is an obligation to care for emergently ill patients. With respect to potential patients it seems that although there is a strong presumption that supports the physician's prerogative to choose whether to initiate a patient-physician relationship it can be superseded by an obligation to treat in specific circumstances. "Physicians cannot refuse to care for patients based on race, gender, sexual orientation, or any other criteria that would constitute invidious discrimination nor can they discriminate against patients with infectious diseases. Physicians may not refuse to care for patients when operating under a contractual arrangement that requires them to treat" [9].

Noncompliance does not excuse physicians from this specific obligation to accept potential patients, nor is it recognized to excuse them from principle 7, which applies to an established patient: "A physician shall, while caring for a patient, regard responsibility to the patient as paramount" [8]. Absent some specific obligation, such as those mentioned previously, however, the code states that physicians have the option of withdrawing from a case without mention of reasons. They should not neglect the patient, however, and they should not do so suddenly. "Physicians have an obligation to support continuity of care for their patients. While physicians have the option of withdrawing from a case, they cannot do so without giving notice to the patient, the relatives, or responsible friends sufficiently long in advance of withdrawal to permit another medical attendant to be secured" [10].

The AMA Code is cited frequently in legal cases related to professional conduct and violations of it could result in loss of AMA membership. Not all physicians and certainly not all surgeons belong to the AMA, however, and those who do not belong could claim that obligations in the Code do not apply to them. The code is also used by many state licensing boards as a behavioral standard for physicians regardless of AMA membership. A state board may sanction or revoke the license of a physician whose actions violate the code. It is difficult to identify self-imposed professional obligations of doctors without recourse to some type of code. The alternative is to refer to tradition or to turn to external sources, such as public expectation or the law.

Surgeons can refer to a variety of codes generally associated with specialties. Because the American College of Surgeons (ACS) has recently done extensive work on its code it is helpful to explore that code's statements about obligations to patients and the response to noncompliance.

The preamble of the ACS Code of Professional Conduct echoes the antidiscrimination language of the AMA Code, which reflects changes in civil rights and federal law, but it asserts a positive obligation to treat patients with respect and tolerance. The latter does seem relevant to the issue of noncompliance. "The ethical practice of medicine establishes and ensures an environment in which all individuals are treated with respect and tolerance; discrimination or harassment on the basis of age, sexual preference, gender, race, disease, disability, or religion, are proscribed as being inconsistent with the ideals and principles of the American College of Surgeons" [11].

The ACS Code itself, although it does not use the word "obligations," uses the word "responsibilities" and provides a short and incisive list of these with respect to "our patients." The most relevant ones are listed next [12]: "During the continuum of pre-, intra-, and postoperative care we accept responsibilities to:

- Serve as effective advocates for our patients' needs.
- Disclose therapeutic options, including their risks and benefits.
- Be sensitive and respectful of patients, understanding their vulnerability during the perioperative period.
- Acknowledge patients' psychological, social, cultural and spiritual needs."

In the section on competencies of the responsible surgeon five points seem directly related to noncompliance [13]. "A responsible surgeon should demonstrate competence in:

1. Patient Care that is compassionate, appropriate, and effective for the treatment of health problems and the promotion of good health.
2. Medical Knowledge about established and evolving biomedical, clinical, and cognate (for example, epidemiological and social-behavioral) sciences and the application of this knowledge to patient care.
3. Practice-Based Learning and Improvement that involves investigation and evaluation of a surgeon's patient care, appraisal and assimilation of scientific evidence, and improvements in patient care.
4. Interpersonal and Communication Skills that result in effective information exchange and effective interaction with patients, their families, and other health care professionals.
5. Professionalism, as manifested through a commitment to carrying out professional responsibilities, adherence to ethical principles, and sensitivity to a diverse patient population."

In its section on the relation of the surgeon to the patient, the ACS code describes informed consent in terms of the proposed operation, but does not say anything about disclosing or agreeing on what medicines or treatments are required or recommended after it or what behaviors are inconsistent with optimal recovery and outcome. It does say, "When patients agree to an operation conditionally or make demands that are unacceptable to the surgeon; the surgeon may elect to withdraw from the case" [14]. This suggests that if a patient is informed about postoperative recommendations and requirements before an operation and refuses to comply with them, this could be regarded as an informed refusal to proceed or an ethical basis for the surgeon to withdraw or at least not to proceed with that particular treatment strategy. An alternative approach might be mutually acceptable to patient and surgeon.

It seems that although physicians are generally free to choose their patients, a person's emergent condition creates a duty to treat. Discrimination toward several identified classes or one's own contractual obligation precludes refusal to treat. Surgeons may have an ethical basis to decline nonemergent care if a potential patient indicates unwillingness to comply with essential postoperative treatments. Once doctors and surgeons, in particular, are in a relationship with a patient, there are obligations or responsibilities to treat that patient competently, respectfully, and tolerantly and not to neglect them. Physicians and surgeons, however, seem to be free to disengage from care for many reasons as long as they provide for actual or possible continuity of care if that is needed and desired by the patient.

Personal obligations to patients are just that. They can exist or be believed for many reasons. Membership in an extended family or a community may confer such an obligation. Training, specialty traditions, or even a particular role model or mentor may foster a special sense of obligation to all or a particular group of patients. A clinician's place in their medical career may alter their sense of obligation to patients and ability and opportunity to meet those obligations.

Personal obligations may stem from a deeply held spiritual or religious conviction. A passage from the Gospel of Saint Luke is a frequently cited example of such a conviction: "From everyone to whom much has been given, much will be required" (Luke 12:48). It is probably worth recalling for those who know it, and noting for those who do not, that Luke was a physician. Sacred texts are replete not only with obligations but with examples of noncompliance, albeit outside the medical domain. They provide a full spectrum of responses to noncompliance. The responses range from lethal punishment to forgiveness and re-education. Noncompliance with religious practice or law is not the same as medical noncompliance, so one should be cautious before formulating a response based on nonanalagous situations.

What is meant and known about medical noncompliance?

Noncompliance, when it is used to describe behavior, generally denotes failure to follow an order, policy, or law. The implication is that the party whose behavior is in question has a legal, contractual, or contextual obligation to conform. Medical patients do not necessarily have this obligation. They have the prerogative to accept or reject medical recommendations for medical treatment, surgery, or changes in habits or behaviors. If they reject these recommendations, however, there may be serious consequences to their health and financial consequences to themselves and to others. Those others may also feel disrespect, disappointment, anger, frustration, and a sense of wasted effort or futility. The emotional reactions are intensified if patients fail to follow or adhere to recommendations or instructions to which they explicitly or tacitly agreed. It may be more accurate and helpful to physicians to identify this behavior as nonadherent because it clarifies that it is a departure from the patient's previous intent rather than a breach of a duty or an obligation to the physician.

Nonadherence is a prevalent human behavior. Just think of unfulfilled New Year's resolutions or health club memberships that go unused. The earliest physicians probably recognized medical nonadherence. Hippocrates wrote, "Keep watch also on the fault of patients which often make them lie about the taking of things prescribed" [15]. Nonadherence with medical regimens is quite common and has been documented to be about 50% with antihypertensive and even antituberculous therapy [16,17]. It has probably grown more common with the advent of drugs that are expensive, require multiple daily doses, and have unpleasant or dangerous side effects. Solid organ transplantation is an excellent example of the challenges that contemporary medical technology and surgery poses for patient adherence. Studies show that nonadherence with immunosuppressive therapy is common: 2% to 68% [18] for all organs and an average of 22% for kidney transplants [19]. Not surprisingly, it is associated with decreased graft survival and increased morbidity.

Although nonadherence is frequent, physicians generally presume adherence and fail to identify most nonadherent patients [20–22]. When they do identify such patients they often think of them as deviant or careless. It may be useful to acknowledge that clinicians too are often nonadherent and even noncompliant. In a hospital-based observational study of physicians' routine hand hygiene practices, Pittet and coworkers [23] found adherence averaged 57% and varied markedly across medical specialties. In multivariate analysis, adherence was associated with the awareness of being observed, the belief of being a role model for other colleagues, a positive attitude toward hand hygiene after patient contact, and easy access to hand-rub solution. Conversely, high workload, activities associated with a high risk for cross-transmission, and certain technical medical specialties (surgery, anesthesiology, emergency medicine, and intensive care medicine) were risk factors for nonadherence.

As that study of physician behavior shows, adherence or nonadherence is complex and multifactorial. Among patients, causes for nonadherence include misunderstanding; inability to comply (financial, physical, or physiologic); and not understanding the reason for a prescription or an action [15,24].

Predicting who is or will be nonadherent is perhaps even more complex and mostly counterintuitive. Poverty and poor education are not predictors. Age, gender, type of disease, and physician sociodemographic characteristics are weak and inconsistent predictors [15,21]. There are psychologic factors that do influence adherence but they are not fixed or easily identified before an illness or injury. They are situational and responsive. They include patients' levels of anxiety; motivation to recover; attitudes toward illness, treatment, and doctor; and the attitudes and beliefs of others including doctors in their environment [15].

When and why is nonadherence relevant?

Surgeons can respond differently to nonadherence if they identify it as an issue before they establish a relationship or operate, than if it occurs in the postoperative period. For example, if a patient refuses blood transfusion for an elective operation the surgeon can agree, perhaps alter the plan, explain the incumbent risks, acknowledge possible benefits, or arrange or suggest a referral to another more experienced or more willing surgeon. If a patient has a behavior or an addiction that could compromise the benefits of surgery, such as organ transplant, the surgeon and team could recommend changes, provide assistance in making them, and require a period of demonstrated adherence before proceeding with surgery. A recent history of nonadherence or addiction before a complex surgical procedure is worrisome, but not sufficient to preclude a patient from consideration. Many patients without that history prove to be nonadherent. Patients with that history who become adherent before surgery demonstrate some of the attitudinal and motivational factors that are associated with sustained adherence. Careful psychologic testing of all prospective transplant patients, not presumptive or stereotypical judgments, although not yet regarded as predictive may prove useful as a factor in counseling or selection [25,26]. Because donor organs are such a scarce resource, it seems justified to make anticipated adherence a criterion for eligibility. Because the consequences of ineligibility are so grave, however, judgment about adherence must be as careful, objective, and accurate as possible.

When nonadherence occurs after an operation, the surgeon faces different problems and has different strategies to use. Because not all nonadherence necessitates another operation, the medical response could come from clinicians responsible for some other aspect of the patient's care, such as cardiologists, infectious disease specialists, or transplant nurse-coordinators. If another operation is necessary but nonurgent and the patient desires it, the surgeon can use the strategies for preoperative nonadherence plus explore the reasons and circumstances that led to this result. Just as not all bad surgical outcomes result from surgeons' nonadherence to standards, not all bad outcomes result from patient nonadherence, even when it occurs. An operative site infection, intravenous catheter infection, or even donor organ failure may occur in a nonadherent patient but not because of the nonadherence. It is important to make the distinction, because patients who feel blamed for what they do not feel responsible for are likely to lose respect and trust in their physician, a critical factor for future adherence. If nonadherence clearly led to the need for surgery it is important to make that connection for the patient. It is equally important to investigate the reasons for it. If the patient was unable to purchase the requisite drugs, it does seem pointless to pursue a second procedure without resolving that problem, which may require the help of other professionals. If the patient has relapsed with an addiction, additional assistance and a period of abstinence are appropriate prerequisites to more surgery.

A particularly vexing problem for thoracic surgeons and for infectious disease physicians is a patient who uses illicit intravenous drugs and who has bacterial endocarditis. Although disturbing, this unlawful behavior, which really is noncompliant, does not excuse a surgeon from an obligation to perform a medically necessary operation. As has been seen, the obligation may not be generic, but it may arise from emergent circumstances, an established relationship, or a contractual commitment. An unobligated surgeon may still choose to proceed with surgery because he or she realizes that noncompliance with the law does not alter the grave prognosis of the infection or necessarily predict nonadherence or a poor surgical result. Studies on patients who are advised to seek help and overcome addictions show that, whereas some predictably fail or relapse, many succeed, in large part because of the factors mentioned previously and the assistance and encouragement of the medical team [25,27,28]. Surgeons often operate on presumed adherent patients with a disease, such as lung cancer, with a lower predicted 5-year survival than a valve replacement in an illicit drug user. The prognosis for the drug user is also more likely to reflect the skill and attitude of the team. Surgeons who decline to operate on such patients should be clear about their reasons and not confuse dislike or distaste for a patient or his or her behavior with a medical contraindication for surgery or with evidence that the surgery will certainly fail. They should also be clear about whether their medical concerns are short-term (ie, perioperative) or long-term, such as recurrent disease or other addiction-related problems. Evidence from patients with addictions to tobacco, alcohol, and illegal drugs may be helpful in this regard [25,27,29].

Does the surgeon have a special obligation to the nonadherent patient?

Because nonadherence is so common, so consequential, and so influenced by physicians, responsible surgeons have an incentive if not a duty to predict, prevent, identify, and manage it. Doing those things well reduces frustrations and produces better outcomes.

Prediction, although not precise, is better than prejudice or intuition. A history of nonadherence to a previous medical regimen, especially a similar one, is certainly a basis for concern. The concerned surgeon should share that concern directly and work with the patient and other professionals to establish and then reduce the risk of nonadherence or, if appropriate, postpone or cancel an operation.

Prevention by selection is a poor tool because there are few, if any, directly observable characteristics that allow a surgeon to screen out nonadherent patients. Prevention is also largely a function of the surgeon. Misunderstanding is preventable, but only if it is anticipated and identified early. Surgeons must communicate clearly and adapt to individual needs and abilities. Professional translators, support persons, written instructions, and pictures all help with understanding. The question, "do you understand," often does not help. If patients can explain to the clinician what they should do and why, then they understand. Otherwise one cannot know whether they understand. Prevention also depends on the surgeon's knowledge of the other essential elements of adherence: ability to pay, ability and means to get to treatment and appointments, and support persons who understand what is expected and are willing and able to help. If any of these elements are missing, steps to correct them may well prevent nonadherence.

Identifying nonadherence can be a challenge. There are false-negatives and false-positives. Clinicians overestimate adherence and often make unsupported assumptions about nonadherence. Unfortunately, if patients are asked about their adherence or are accused of nonadherence, they are being invited to lie. If it is acknowledged that adherence is hard for everyone and that at least some difficulty with complicated regimens is expected, an atmosphere in which it may be easier for some nonadherent patients to tell the truth is created. One should suspect, but not presume, nonadherence when the clinical course is not what is expected. Although other possibilities are pursued, it may be useful to have patients bring in their prescriptions to be sure they are correct, that they are labeled properly, to see how many pills have been taken, and when the prescription was filled. A physical examination for signs of tobacco or drug use and laboratory tests can be helpful when addiction is the concern.

Managing nonadherence may not be a technical skill acquired in training, or one that wins accolades from colleagues, but it can be the difference between a good surgeon or program as measured by outcomes and excellent ones. An article by the surgeon Gawande [30] makes that point about programs that treat cystic fibrosis. I suspect the same is true of heart transplant programs.

Summary

Professional oaths and codes do not establish a firm basis for the obligation to treat all patients and they provide little or no clear guidance about whether patient nonadherence exempts a physician from a specific contextual obligation to a patient. A long-standing and still prevalent tradition in surgery supports a strong obligation to one's established patients. A personal belief in an obligation to serve those less fortunate or even less compliant could support sustained treatment and special assistance to a nonadherent patient. A collective, professional, objective, informed decision to exclude a patient who is highly likely to be nonadherent or incapable of adherence from the benefit of a scarce resource, such as a human organ, is defensible and appropriate. A surgeon's decision to deny care to an established but nonadherent patient is much less so. Adherence is as dependent on physician attitude, skill, and behavior as it is on patients' nonadherence. To the degree that it reflects less than competent management of this prevalent problem, it can be considered an error or complication that makes most surgeons feel even more obliged to mitigate or rectify the problem. This article describes the almost ubiquitous phenomenon of nonadherence; a way to reconceptualize noncompliance; and practical steps that can help predict, prevent, identify, and manage it. It is hoped that this helps surgeons reduce the frequency of nonadherence, make dealing with it less onerous, and consequently achieve better outcomes.

It is reasonable to think about nonadherence in terms of three roles. The surgeon's role is to make the patient's choice informed, to be aware of the risk factors for nonadherence, and not make adherence any more difficult than it has to be. The patient's role is to make choices between value-laden alternatives. Society's role is equitably to distribute scarce medical resources to patients who can and want to adhere to the necessary regimen to benefit from them [31].

Acknowledgments

Linda Carr-Lee and Natalie Burbank provided valuable research and editorial assistance and manuscript preparation.

References

[1] Edelstein L. Translation from the Greek. In: Edelstein L, editor. The Hippocratic Oath: text, translation, and interpretation. Baltimore: Johns Hopkins Press; 1943.
[2] Gabriel BA. Oath of Lasagna (1964). In: A Hippocratic Oath for our time. American Association of Medical Colleges. September 2001. Available at: www.aamc.org/newsroom/reporter/sept2001/hippocraticoath.htm. Accessed May 28, 2005.
[3] The Oath of Maimonides. In: Halsall P, editor. Internet history sourcebooks project. Available at: http://www.fordham.edu/halsall/source/rambam-oath.html.Accessed May 28, 2005.
[4] Gabriel BA. Declaration of Geneva (World Medical Association 1948). In: A Hippocratic Oath for our time. American Association of Medical Colleges. September 2001. Available at: www.aamc.org/newsroom/reporter/sept2001/hippocraticoath.htm. Accessed May 28, 2005.
[5] Gabriel BA. A Hippocratic Oath for Our Time. American Association of Medical Colleges. September 2001. Available at: www.aamc.org/newsroom/reporter/sept2001/hippocraticoath.htm. Accessed May 28, 2005.
[6] American Medical AssociationCode of Ethics, adopted May, 1847. Philadelphia: Turner-Hamilton; 1871.
[7] Council on Ethical and Judicial Affairs. Code of Medical Ethics: Current opinions with annotations. American Medical Association: 2002: 286. Available at: http://www.ama-assn.org/ama/pub/category/2498.html. Accessed May 28, 2005.

[8] Council on Ethical and Judicial Affairs. Code of Medical Ethics: Current opinions with annotations. American Medical Association: 2002: XIV. Available at: http://www.ama-assn.org/ama/pub/category/2512.html. Accessed May 28, 2005.

[9] Council on Ethical and Judicial Affairs. Code of Medical Ethics: Current opinions with annotations. American Medical Association: 2002: 289. Available at: http://www.ama-assn.org/ama/pub/category/2512.html. Accessed May 28, 2005.

[10] Council on Ethical and Judicial Affairs. Code of Medical Ethics: Current opinions with annotations. American Medical Association: 2002: 217. Available at: http://www.ama-assn.org/ama/pub/category/2512.html. Accessed May 28, 2005.

[11] American College of Surgeons, preamble. Avaliable at: http://www.facs.org/fellows_info/statements/stonprin.html#pre. Accessed May 28, 2005.

[12] American College of Surgeons, Code of Professional Conduct. Available at: http://www.facs.org/fellows_info/statements/stonprin.html#pre. Accessed May 28, 2005.

[13] American College of Surgeons, Qualifications of the Responsible Surgeon, Competencies. Available at: http://www.facs.org/fellows_info/statements/stonprin.html#pre. Accessed May 28, 2005.

[14] American College of Surgeons, Relation of the Surgeon to the Patient. Available at: http://www.facs.org/fellows_info/statements/stonprin.html#pre. Accessed May 28, 2005.

[15] Evans L, Spelman M. The problem of non-compliance with drug therapy. Drugs 1983;25: 63–76.

[16] Costa FV. Compliance with anti-hypertensive treatment. Clin Exp Hypertens 1996;18: 463–72.

[17] Dixon WM, Stradling P, Woolton DP. Outpatient PAS therapy. Lancet 1957;2:871–2.

[18] Butler JA, Roderick P, Mullee M, et al. Frequency and impact of nonadherence to immuno-suppressants after renal transplantation: a systematic review. Transplantation 2004;77: 769–76.

[19] Chisholm MA. Issues of adherence to immunosuppressant therapy after solid-organ transplantation. Drugs 2002;62:567–75.

[20] Wright EC. Non-compliance—or how many ants has Matilda? Lancet 1993;342:909–13.

[21] Stephenson BJ, Rowe BH, Haynes RB, et al. Is this patient taking the treatment as prescribed? JAMA 1993;269:2779–81.

[22] Melinkow J, Kiefe C. Patient compliance and medical research: issues in methodology. J Gen Intern Med 1994;9:96–105.

[23] Pittet D, Simon A, Hugonnet S, et al. Hand hygiene among physicians: performance, beliefs, and perceptions. Ann Intern Med 2004;141:1–8.

[24] Fletcher RH. Patient compliance with therapeutic advice: a modern view. Mt Sinai J Med 1989;56:453–8.

[25] Maxson PM, Schultz KL, Berge KH, et al. Probable alcohol abuse or dependence: a risk factor for intensive-care readmission in patients undergoing elective vascular and thoracic surgical procedures. May Perioperative Outcomes Group. Mayo Clin Proc 1999;74:448–53.

[26] Shapiro PA, Williams DL, Foray AT, et al. Psychosocial evaluation and prediction of compliance problems and morbidity after heart transplantation. Transplantation 1995;60: 1462–6.

[27] Dresler CM, Bailey M, Roper CR, et al. Smoking cessation and lung cancer resection. Chest 1996;110:1199–202.

[28] Bellamy CO, DiMartini AM, Ruppert K, et al. Liver transplantation for alcoholic cirrhosis: long term follow-up and impact of disease recurrence. Transplantation 2001;72:619–26.

[29] Hanrahan JS, Eberly C, Mohanty PK. Substance abuse in heart transplant recipients: a 10-year follow-up study. Prog Transplant 2001;11:285–90.

[30] Gawande A. The bell curve: what happens when patients find out how good their doctors really are. The New Yorker December 6, 2004;80:82–95.

[31] Jacobson JA. Compliance and adherence. In: Sugarman J, editor. Twenty common problems: ethics in primary care. New York: McGraw-Hill; 2000. p. 39–48.

ELSEVIER
SAUNDERS

SURGICAL
CLINICS OF
NORTH AMERICA

Surg Clin N Am 87 (2007) 949–960

The Global Impact of Surgical Volunteerism

Kathleen M. Casey, MD, FACS

American College of Surgeons, Operation Giving Back,
633 N. Saint Clair Street, Chicago, IL 60611, USA

> You must give some time to your fellow man. For remember, you don't live in a world all your own. Your brothers are here too.
> —Albert Schweitzer, MD

Surgeons have a proud tradition of responding to societal needs beyond their classic role as caregivers to individual patients. Whether active in local communities or global initiatives, surgical volunteers experience a profound sense of meaning that resonates with the altruistic roots of the surgical profession.

Beyond its transformative effect on providers and recipients, it is fair to ask some fundamental questions about volunteer care. What is the significance of volunteerism to what might be called the overall surgical industry? Can volunteerism shape systems, societies, and economies? Often considered little more than a collection of small-scale enterprises, the magnitude and potential influence of the volunteer sector is still not fully appreciated. Until recently, existing analyses did not accurately reflect the economic impact of the voluntary and nonprofit sectors. However, there is both qualitative and quantitative evidence that illustrates the magnitude of impact of surgical volunteerism.

Assessing the scope of the voluntary and nonprofit sector

A robust method for assessing the scope of the voluntary and nonprofit sector has been jointly developed by the Johns Hopkins Center for Civil Society Studies and the United Nations Statistics Division. Their initial study of 30 countries confirms "what many people already suspected: that nonprofit organizations and volunteering constitute a massive economic force" [1]. In

E-mail address: kcasey@facs.org

doi:10.1016/j.suc.2007.07.018

fact, the nonprofit and volunteer sector in the United States has been growing at a rate exceeding that of the overall GDP by 20% [1] and is larger than the agriculture, construction, transportation, and utilities sectors [2].

Such economic magnitude carries with it significant influence in the realms of policy, partnerships, and practices. The voluntary sector possesses unique flexibility to respond to perceived gaps in services provided by existing governmental and institutional programs. It also possesses tremendous potential energy and catalytic power in the dedication, imagination, and entrepreneurship of its constituency. It is increasingly apparent that addressing the "serious global social and economic problems that plague our communities will require...the ingenuity and initiative of the world's growing nonprofit sector and the millions of volunteers it can help mobilize. They have the ability to extend the Government's reach, engage grass-roots energies, build cross-sector partnerships and reinvigorate democratic governance" [1]. Understanding the dynamic power of this sector provides context for the important role that volunteer surgeons play.

The role of surgeons in the voluntary and nonprofit sector

In examining the role and contributions of surgeons in the nonprofit/voluntary sector, the bulk of activity occurs on the international stage. Historically, major humanitarian efforts have been undertaken in foreign lands, with thousands of medical nonprofit organizations providing services ranging in nature from education to clinical medicine to telemedicine and other emerging technologies. No less than two dozen initiatives successful in providing surgical care, education, training, and needed supplies have been founded by member surgeons of the American College of Surgeons.

These considerable accomplishments are significant, not only to individuals and communities served, but also on a personal and professional level to those providing care. For every hospital built in a community once lacking health care, the resulting benefits extend beyond providing care for local citizens to professional training, economic growth potential, and infrastructure to support healthy communities. For every training program implemented to help eradicate debilitating congenital or acquired surgical conditions, individuals, systems, and communities are transformed. For every international partnership established, generations of collaboration and exchange are possible.

Measuring positive impact and demonstrating lasting effect has been a challenge for the nonprofit sector. Because of a perceived lack of meaningful gauges of effectiveness of nonprofit efforts, there is growing interest in defining and applying measures of the impact and sustainability of humanitarian work. The Sphere Project, an international initiative established in 1997 in Geneva, Switzerland, has developed a *Humanitarian Charter and Minimum Standards in Disaster Response* dedicated to improving the effectiveness and accountability of disaster response, with a focus on what those affected by disasters have a right to expect from humanitarian aid [3].

The Humanitarian Accountability Partnership (HAP), also Geneva-based, was implemented in 2003 to make "humanitarian action accountable to beneficiaries" by means of an international self-regulatory body that monitors, guides, and supports nonprofit humanitarian programs. HAP provides certificates to those programs that adhere to defined standards and practices [4].

The University of Washington recently announced the launch of the Institute for Health Metrics and Evaluation with a $105 million grant from the Gates Foundation [5]. Their stated mission is to "guide international policy-making" using high-quality data on needs and outcomes analyses [4]. Examining what works and trying to determining the portability of effective programs to different cultures, economies, or climates are positive steps forward. The increased scrutiny and attention to benchmarking should greatly enhance the mission and efficacy of existing efforts.

As each community in need presents a different combination of resources, politics, challenges, and opportunities, a spectrum of responses is both valid and appropriate. While no simple solutions exist, several elements are always appropriate, whether volunteering in the United States or abroad. These include cultural sensitivity, mutual respect, well-managed expectations, and partnership with those served. An appreciation of the role of long-term relationships is essential in effecting sustainable change. In an ideal world, volunteer outreach pursuits would consist of true partnerships working toward sustainable solutions to identified problems, which ultimately would obviate the need for the volunteer effort. In the real world, of course, political, social, economic, religious, and practical issues intervene.

The recent work of Salamon and colleagues in assessing the economic significance of the voluntary sector raises the question of whether the proper measurement tools have yet been identified for assessing true impact. Are we examining these issues through the proper lens?

Examining the impact of the voluntary and nonprofit sector

Touted as a collateral benefit of medical outreach with deeply important consequences, the concept of *medical diplomacy* recently has been emphasized. The nonprofit organization, Terror Free Tomorrow, has examined the impact of American humanitarian leadership in potentially "hostile" regions. Their work has demonstrated that outreach to countries in need, as in Indonesia following the 2004 tsunamis or after Pakistan's devastating earthquake in 2005, has had sustainable impact not only in reversing negative attitudes towards the US but also decreasing popular support for global terrorists [6].

After the tsunami, the hospital ship USNS Mercy was deployed to the region with a combined crew of military and volunteer medical staff from the nonprofit organization Project HOPE. After a follow-up mission to the region, a 2006 survey conducted in Indonesia and Bangladesh, the world's largest and third largest Muslim countries respectively, demonstrated a 63% favorable response to the humanitarian medical mission of the USNS Mercy among Indonesians, and a 95% favorable response among Bangladeshis [6]. Not only did this mission favorably change public opinion towards the United States, but also the "consensus approval of the Mercy mission cut across every demographic and political view" [7]. In a similar fashion, Terror Free Tomorrow concluded that 78% of Paistanis had a more favorable opinion of the United States because of American earthquake relief [8]. "Importantly, this change in perception lasted beyond the initial aid and service, underscoring that America's actions can have a lasting impact" [9].

The Pentagon's Joint Chiefs of Staff conclude in *The National Military Strategic Plan for the War on Terrorism* that American humanitarian assistance is "often key to demonstrating benevolence and goodwill abroad...[and] countering ideological support for terrorism" [8]. Understanding the correlation between political unrest, economic instability, and poor health, the significance of these interventions is further magnified. A Brookings Institute policy group observed, "The role of international volunteer service in building bridges across growing global divides has never been more critical to the future of our nation, and global peace and stability" [9].

Other initiatives leading to sustained impact include contributions to the medical education, medical infrastructure, and medical economics of developing countries. Academic partnerships such as the Touch Foundation, which joins the Weill Cornell Medical College with the Bugando University College of Health Sciences in Mwanza, Tanzania, represent long-term commitment to collaboration [10]. Additional global health initiatives fostering international exchange have been established by the medical schools at Brown University, the University of California, San Francisco (UCSF), Johns Hopkins, the University of Colorado, New York University, and others. These academic partnerships have placed a focus on teaching and training directed to local needs and resources. The Pan African Academy of Christian Surgeons has implemented general surgical residency programs in Sub-Saharan Africa in collaboration with Loma Linda Medical University. Oversight is provided by the West African College of Surgeons and the College of Surgeons of East, Central, and Southern Africa.

The needs at home

> The only real nation is humanity.
> —Paul Farmer, MD

Some may question why most medical outreach occurs in countries other than our own. The striking disparity of resources between the United States and other countries provides some insight. Half the world's population lives on less than $2 a day. Tanzania has only two physicians for every 100,000 people, as compared with 256 for every 100,000 people in the United States [11]. This parallels a widespread lack of access to care in many developing nations.

These facts do not obviate the unmet patients' needs that continue to exist in the United States. With nearly 45 million uninsured in the United States who have limited access to nonemergent care, administering appropriate and timely surgical care to this cohort is a challenging situation. The question of how to provide medical care for the underserved is decidedly different than how to provide surgical care.

Much that occurs on the international stage can inform and enhance the delivery of care in the United States. Surgeons volunteering internationally return to their own communities with enhanced awareness of cultural influences on health and a sensitivity to the economic importance of allocating limited resources. Such returning travelers can better appreciate the way our United States systems operate and envision the possibility of providing local care with less elaborate support systems.

Still, most surgeons find it easier to volunteer outside the United States than within it. Liability, licensing, and logistical considerations complicate the provision of humanitarian care in the United States, especially with the wide variations resulting from different state regulations.

Another consideration for surgeons and others who perform procedural care in the United States, is that most of them cannot provide that care within the system of free clinics, because of how they are designed currently. The dependence on an appropriate facility in which to operate, and collaboration with the entire team needed to administer preoperative, interoperative, postoperative, and follow-up care, increase the level of complexity for surgical outreach. Effective delivery of surgical care to this population requires coordinated donation of the spectrum of services from all members of the surgical team and is contingent on committed support from the hospitals or surgi-centers where such care can be provided.

In May 2007, *Health Affairs* reported that "uninsured patients and those who pay with their own funds are charged 2.5 times more for hospital care than those covered by health insurance and more than 3 times the allowable amount paid by Medicare" [12]. Thus, it is easily understood how a "routine" outpatient operation for a hernia or a torn meniscus would be financially devastating. Being uninsured in the United States means receiving less care and less timely care.

Innovative solutions

Several innovative programs created by surgeons have addressed the issue of providing outpatient surgical care to uninsured patients, with strikingly similar solutions. Central in each is partnership with the administration of a local hospital or outpatient surgical clinic in delivering this humanitarian care. By leveraging the relative availability of hospital operating rooms on weekends and benefiting from altruistic volunteers across the spectrum of surgical care providers, each has arrived at an arrangement appropriate for their hospital and tailored to their community's needs and resources.

Operation Access [13] uses operating rooms available on weekends in 19 hospitals in the greater San Francisco area to provide outpatient, elective surgical care to the working poor. In existence since 1993, it now serves patients from 60 community clinics and draws on the services of over 400 health care volunteers. In 2006, Operation Access provided $1.3 million in donated surgical care.

Surgery on Sunday, a similar program in Lexington, Kentucky, donates a full spectrum of outpatient surgical care one Sunday a month. The organization has met with such success in its first year that it is in the process of replicating its plan in other regions of Kentucky [14].

Fresh Start Surgical Gifts in San Diego has been integrating surgical care, surgical training for providers, and research into its Surgery Weekends since 1991 to provide disadvantaged children and young adults with corrective surgery for birth defects, accidents, abuse, or disease. Over the course of seven Surgery Weekends in 2006, Fresh Start delivered $1.4 million in reconstructive surgery and related medical services [15].

Mission Cataract USA demonstrates another innovative approach to serving the uninsured in one's own community. It aids ophthalmologists in establishing designated cataract days when the uninsured can benefit from donated cataract operations [16].

Several common themes characterize these programs. Foremost, they have reframed the central issue: uninsured patients exist in every community, and they will need surgical care. Establishing a mechanism to proactively provide donated care transforms the burden of uncompensated care into an intentional humanitarian act which both honors and respects the patients and the care team. By designating "surgery days", the donated care is quantifiable and provides a concrete demonstration of a deep commitment to community. And, at least theoretically, providing this care in an elective fashion prevents late presentations of surgical conditions and diseases, eliminating the downstream expense of neglected surgical conditions. The organizations above demonstrate volunteerism's potential to transform systems of care and positively impact societal and economic issues.

A vast and largely untapped resource for domestic medical volunteerism is the estimated 160,000 retired surgeons and physicians in the United States. A widely expressed sentiment among this constituency is a reluctance to leave practice altogether, despite limited options for remaining clinically active. Provided with the proper opportunities, licensing, credentialing mechanisms, and charitable immunity protection, this cohort constitutes an enormously powerful force. The Volunteers in Medicine Institute [17] and the American Health Initiative's TAP-IN [18] are programs that recognize and capitalize on this experience pool to care for the uninsured in communities across the United States. Unique constraints still apply to retired surgeons who need hospital operating privileges to do more than diagnose surgical conditions.

Volunteers in times of disaster

Knowing is not enough; we must apply. Willing is not enough; we must do.
— Johann Wolfgang von Goethe

Potential avenues that enable volunteers to provide surgical care for the domestic uninsured may be gleaned from the process of establishing our response to future domestic disasters. Recent natural and human-made disasters have focused a spotlight on the inefficiencies and obstacles in our current system of response. The need for health care providers to cross state lines to provide relief in a disaster or emergency seems obvious in the wake of these events. So, too, is a scalable response system that can draw from a pool of situationally appropriate disaster responders to provide surge capacity.

Most hospitals, communities, and states have disaster plans, but ensuring that they complement and work in concert with each other is paramount for maximal effectiveness. Collaboration with local, regional, national, and international government agencies, the military, and nongovernmental agencies involved in disaster response is essential. More fundamentally, necessary legal avenues must be established that enable health care providers to contribute care appropriate to the situation and their level of proficiency. In late 2006, the National Conference of Commissioners on Uniform State Laws drafted *The Uniformed Emergency Volunteer Health Practitioners Act*, which proposed a legal means of facilitating the interstate deployment of health practitioners "while still allowing host states to act when necessary to limit, restrict, and regulate the use of volunteer health practitioners within their boundaries" [19]. Compared to existing Emergency Management Assistance Compact mutual aid agreements, this proposal incorporates private sector health providers into state forces rather than enabling only government employees to cross state lines in emergency response. In addition, this comprehensive proposal examines definitions of volunteers, volunteer registration systems, credentialing, liability, and other critical considerations.

If such disaster plans and legislation are established in a broad enough manner, the licensing, credentialing, and liability provisions put in place to protect patients and providers in disasters could be modified for application in everyday circumstances. This would lay the necessary groundwork to enable surgeons and other care providers to volunteer to address the less sensational problems of the uninsured.

By volunteering in their own communities, surgeons also gain a greater awareness of existing community medical assets, how they complement each other, and what resources and partnerships may still be needed. In the case of a sudden loss of usual infrastructure in a disaster or emergency, the informal networks of the volunteer community may prove critical for identifying appropriate individuals for a surge capacity group familiar with alternate strategies for delivering care.

The educational value of volunteerism

The next generation of surgeons, while meeting needs locally, must also take a leadership role globally—the need for international partnership has never been greater.

—Doruk Ozgediz, MD

There is a groundswell of understanding, interest, and action in surgical volunteerism. This is especially apparent in the emerging generation of health care providers. Increasingly, students entering medical school have international volunteer experience and an avid interest in global health issues. Opportunities abound for students to nurture this interest during medical school with greater availability of global health programs and formal international elective opportunities. In addition, 52% of medical schools have opportunities for outreach in the local community by means of student-run clinics for the uninsured [20].

This passion finds few formal outlets in surgical residency, as there is a paucity of organized opportunities to participate in volunteer outreach. The complexities are well recognized—an 80-hour work week, logistics, costs, liability and safety concerns, and oversight of educational experience.

Balancing these concerns is the assertion that participation in volunteer medical experiences will enrich resident education in concrete and abstract ways. In considering optimal educational outcomes, volunteer experiences provide many learning opportunities that appear to ideally complement clinical rotations and didactic sessions. There is the potential to increase cultural sensitivity, gain a broader perspective of the American health care system, develop experiential insights on the influence of resource allocation on global health issues, and be exposed to a different spectrum of pathology. Resourcefulness and critical thinking skills that come from working without the benefits of a well-equipped American hospital are difficult, if not impossible, to replicate in the current training paradigm. Arguably, such skills will be required for leaders of the health care systems of the future.

Proven models

An international one month elective in Kenya has been in place for 9 years for general surgery residents at Brown Medical School. A retrospective study was recently conducted to assess the perceived educational, professional, and social growth of participants from the first eight years.

From the perspective of participants, fellow residents, and faculty, those residents who took part in the Kenya elective were noted to demonstrate improved physical examination and decision-making skills, greater cost-effectiveness, and a sense of having returned "a better doctor." It was also learned that many residents had sought out Brown University's surgery program because such an elective was offered. Among faculty, 97% believed the elective to be a valuable component of surgical education for those involved, and 74% would participate in the international volunteer experience if given the opportunity (Klaristenfeld DD, Chupp M, Cioffi WG, and colleagues, unpublished manuscript, 2007).

Residents in the UCSF Orthopedics program have also had access to an international elective since 1992. Participants have consistently rated this experience as the most meaningful of their training, and most continue to participate in volunteer activities following residency [21]. Based on the enthusiasm and benefits seen with their orthopedic colleagues, the general surgery residents at UCSF are currently developing a similar program in Uganda [22].

Among surgical residents, there is a wealth of initiative, passion, and commitment to health care for the underserved in our country and others. At least two nonprofit organizations have been started by surgeons during their residencies. Doug Burka, MD founded the Carefree Foundation to address treatable conditions in underserved populations, and create "treatment environments that foster hope" [23]. Awori Hayanga, MD established the Ruben J. Williams Foundation to address disparities in the provision of surgical care in developing countries with a specific emphasis on Eastern Africa, and a focus on education and training [24].

The role of the American College of Surgeons

> By giving of your time and heart, you will not only help to advance the humane practice of surgery, but you will also reap the rewards of belonging to the greatest humanitarian profession in the world.
> —Kathryn Anderson, MD, FACS

Humanitarian instincts and actions are deeply ingrained in surgeons' professional identity. Sir William Osler noted, "Medicine arose out of the primal sympathy of man with man; out of the desire to help those in sorrow, need and sickness" [25]. This "primal sympathy" and a sense of professional duty motivate many surgeons to offer their services *gratis* to those most in need in their own community or within the global community. Thousands of years ago, Hippocrates, author of our professional oath, acknowledged this as well: "Sometimes give of your services for nothing. And if there is an opportunity for serving one who is a stranger in financial straits, give full assistance to all such. For wherever the art of medicine is loved, there is also a love of humanity" [26].

Today, the Code of Professional Conduct of the American College of Surgeons (ACS) echoes these same principles with guidelines advising surgeons to:

> "Provide necessary surgical care without regard to gender, race, disability, religion, social status or ability to pay;
>
> Advocate strategies to improve individual and public health by communicating with government, health care organizations, and industry; and
>
> Work with society to establish just, effective and efficient distribution of health care resources" [27].

The ACS has recognized the magnitude of interest and involvement in surgical volunteerism and is working to make it easier for surgeons to engage in volunteerism at all stages of their careers. The College's volunteer initiative, Operation Giving Back (OGB) was created to recognize, connect, support, enable, and celebrate those surgeons interested in volunteerism. OGB aims to "facilitate surgical volunteerism" for surgeons of all specialties and at all career stages. Facilitating surgical volunteerism is a simple phrase that encompasses a wide and complex scope of intent, related to all of the topics discussed in this article, and others as they are identified. What distinguishes this effort is the tailoring of its resources and database for and by surgeons, and recognition of the unique challenges involved in ensuring adequate surgical care in diverse circumstances. OGB identifies surgeons with an interest in volunteerism and fosters partnership between individuals in academia and private practice, corporations, foundations, and nonprofit entities, looking toward possibilities for synergy and further transformational potential of surgical volunteerism.

> In every community there is work to be done. In every nation there are wounds to heal. In every heart, there is the power to do it.
>
> —Marianne Williamson

The importance of the clinical, societal, political, and economic impact of volunteerism is becoming better appreciated. However, questions remain with regard to providing surgical care to those without adequate means or access. In the end, the most effective mechanisms are sought for translating volunteer interest and effort into meaningful results. Facilitating collaboration among the many individuals and organizations invested in surgical volunteerism will magnify the contributions from the surgical community in caring for the underserved.

The enduring commitment of surgeons to these matters inspires confidence that solutions will continue to come from the surgical community, in keeping with a rich professional legacy. With an emerging generation of surgeons passionate about their ability to give back in a global society, and so many practicing and retired surgeons pursuing similar opportunities to contribute, the time is ripe to foster these interests and actions.

References

[1] Salamon LM. Director of the Johns Hopkins Center for Civil Society Studies, "Putting the Non-profit Sector and Volunteerism on the Economic Map," from United Nations Volunteers. Available at: www.unv.org/en/news-resources/resources/on-volunteerism/doc/the-chronicle-interview.html. Accessed July 5, 2007.

[2] Salamon LM. "New U.N. Guidelines Put Civil Society on the World's Economic Map," from Headlines@Hopkins: Johns Hopkins University News Releases. Available at: www.jhu.edu/news-info/new/home06/sept06/unguide.html. Accessed July 5, 2007.

[3] Sphere Project. Available at: www.sphereproject.org. Accessed July 10, 2007.

[4] Humanitarian Accountability Partnership—International. Available at: www.hapinternational.org. Accessed July 10, 2007.

[5] University of Washington Medical Press Release. Available at: http://www.uwmedicine.org/Global/NewsAndEvents/PressReleases/2006/Gates+Gift+for+Global+Health+Institute.htm. Accessed July 10, 2007.

[6] Terror Free Tomorrow poll. One year later: humanitarian releif sustains change in Muslim public opinion. 2006. Available at: http//www.terrorfreetomorrow.org/upimagestft/INDONESIA%202006%20Poll%20Report.pdf. Accessed July 1, 2007.

[7] Terror Free Tomorrow poll. Unprecedented Terror Free Tomorrow polls: world's largest Muslim countries welcome US navy. 2006. Available at: http://www.terrorfreetomorrow.org/upimagestft/Final%20Mercy%20Poll%20Report.pdf. Accessed July 1, 2007.

[8] Terror Free Tomorrow poll. A dramatic change of public opinion in the Muslim world. 2005. Available at: http://www.terrorfreetomorrow.org/upimagestft/Pakistan%20Poll%20Report-updated.pdf. Accessed July 1, 2007.

[9] Caprara D. The best diplomats: American volunteers, WashingtonPost.com's think tank town. January 7, 2007. Available at: http://www.washingtonpost.com/wp-dyn/content/article/2007/01/07/AR2007010701270.html. Accessed August 8, 2007.

[10] Touch Foundation. Available at: www.touchfoundation.org. Accessed July 9, 2007.

[11] World Health Organization Core Health Indicators, latest available data. Available at: www.who.int/whosis/database/core/core-select.cfm. Accessed July 16, 2007.

[12] Anderson GF. From 'soak the rich' to 'soak the poor': recent trends in hospital pricing. Health Aff (Millwood) 2007;26(3):780–9.

[13] Operation Access, 2006 Annual Report PDF. Available at: http://www.operationaccess.org/pdf/AnnualReport2006.pdf; http://www.operationaccess.org. Accessed July 10, 2007.

[14] Surgery On Sunday. Available at: http://www.surgeryonsunday.org/. Accessed July 10, 2007.

[15] Fresh Start Surgical Gifts, Annual Report PDF. Available at: http://www.freshstart.org/uploads/files/AR2006.pdf; http://www.freshstart.org. Accessed July 10, 2007.

[16] Mission Cataract USA. Available at: http://www.missioncataractusa.org/index.php?n=1&;id=1. Accessed July 10, 2007.

[17] Volunteers in Medicine Institute. Available at: http://www.vimi.org/. Accessed July 10, 2007.

[18] Tap-In. Available at: http://tap-in.org. Accessed July 10, 2007.

[19] Uniformed Emergency Volunteer Health Practitioners Act, drafted by the National Conference of Commissioners on Uniform State Laws. Available at: http://www.law.upenn.edu/bll/archives/ulc/uiehsa/2006act_final.htm. Accessed December 6, 2006 (p.4).

[20] Simpson SA, Long JA. Medical student-run health clinics: important contributors to patient care and medical education. J Gen Intern Med 2007;22(3):352–6.

[21] "'Into Africa' for UCSF Orthopedic Surgery Residents". Available at: http://orthosurg.ucsf.edu/orthotrauma/html/education_int_outreach.htm. Accessed June 19, 2007.

[22] Ozgediz D, Roayaie K, Debas H, et al. Surgery in developing countries: essential training in residency. Arch Surg 2005;140(8):795–800.

[23] The Carefree Foundation. Available at: http://www.carefreefoundation.org/. Accessed July 10, 2007.
[24] Hayanga A. Volunteerism in general surgical residency: fostering sustainable global academic partnerships. Arch Surg 2007;142(6):577–9.
[25] Osler W. In Evolution of Modern Medicine, Chapter II, Manuscript of 1913 lecture delivered at Yale University. New Haven (CT): Yale University Press; 1923.
[26] Hippocrates of Kos, 460 BC-377 BC.
[27] American College of Surgeons Code of Professional Conduct. Available at: http://www.facs.org/memberservices/codeofconduct.html. Accessed July 10, 2007.

**ELSEVIER
SAUNDERS**

Surg Clin N Am 87 (2007) 961–964

SURGICAL
CLINICS OF
NORTH AMERICA

Index

Note: Page numbers of article titles are in **boldface** type.

A

American Board of Medical Specialties, in certification for surgery, 826, 827

American Board of Surgery
and graduate medical education, 821
in certification for surgery, 825
in regulatory oversight, 814–816

American College of Surgeons
and new surgical procedures and technology, 860–861, 864
and physician supply and demand, 806, 808
and surgical volunteerism, 957–958
in assessment of surgical care, 848

American College of Surgeons Code of Professional Conduct, and surgeons' obligations, to noncompliant patients, 940–942

American College of Surgeons reports, on patient access, to surgical workforce, 800

American Medical Association Code of Ethics, and surgeons' obligations, to noncompliant patients, 939–940

Anesthesia, and patient safety, 868

B

Bureau of Health Professions, and physician supply and demand, 798

C

Centers for Medicaid and Medicare Services, in patient safety, 875–876

Certification in surgery, **825–836**
American Board of Medical Specialties and, 826, 827
American Board of Surgery and, 825
benefits of, 834–835
for clinically inactive surgeons, 834

historical aspects of, 825
initial, requirements for, 826–827
Miller's pyramid in, 827
multiple certificates in, 833–834
physician competence and, broader assessment of, 830–833
assessment of practice performance in, 832–833
competencies in, 830–832
components of, 832–833
self-assessment in, 831–832
time-limited, emergence and rationale for, 827–830
fail rates in, 828–829

Computerized physician order entry
and better care, 884
and patient safety, 872

Consent, informed. *See* Informed consent.

Council on Graduate Medical Education, and physician supply and demand, 798, 799–800, 805–806

Crew resource management, in patient safety, 870, 871

Crossover testimony, by expert witnesses, 896–897

E

Emergency Medical Treatment and Active Labor Act, and patient access, to surgical workforce, 803

Employers, as health care purchasers, **883–887**
banding together for greater market force, 883–887
Leapfrog Group and, 883–887
paying for better care, 885–887
return on investment estimator in, 886
pushing for better care, 884–885
computerized physician order entry in, 884

Employers (*continued*)
    evidence-based hospital referral
        in, 885
    intensive care unit physician
        staffing in, 884–885
    Leapfrog Safe Practices Score in,
        885
Expert witnesses, **889–901**
    crossover testimony by, 896–897
    definition of negligence and, 890–891
    differing opinions by, 895–896
    generalists versus specialists, 894–895
    legal system overview and, 889–890
    necessity for, 891
    professional status of, 897–898
    qualifications of, 891–892
    rationale for, 899–900
    standard of care and, 892–894
        geographic issues in, 892–894
    unscrupulous, 898–899

F

Flexner report, on physician supply and
    demand, 798

Fresh Start Surgical Gifts, and surgical
    volunteerism, 954

G

Graduate medical education, **811–823**
    funding for, 813–814
    historical aspects of, 811–813
    issues confronting, 816–823
        attractiveness of surgery as
            career, 816–817
        attrition from residency
            programs, 818
        competency of graduating
            residents, 820
        increasing subspecialization, 818
        limitations on work hours,
            819–820
        response of profession to,
            820–823
            American Board of Surgery,
                821
            assess public need for
                surgeons, 823
            define scope of specialty,
                821–822
            Internet in, 822
            Surgical Council on
                Resident Education,
                821–822
            surgical skills laboratory in,
                822
    regulatory oversight of, 814–816

American Board of Surgery in,
    814–816
Residency Review Committee for
    Surgery in, 815–816
residency programs in, 813
residents' legal status in, 814

Graduate Medical Education National
    Advisory Committee, and physician
    supply and demand, 798

H

Hippocratic Oath, and surgeons'
    obligations, to noncompliant patients,
    938

I

Informed consent, **903–918**
    and surgeons' obligations, to
        noncompliant patients, 941–942
    conflicting professional opinions in,
        912
    disclosure obligations in, 906–907
    documentation of, in medical record,
        908
    for children, 915–916
    for surgery performed by supervised
        trainees, 916
    historical aspects of, 904–905
    in research, 916–917
    patient's understanding of, 907–908
    patients who are undecided or refuse
        surgery, 913–914
    problems with patient's
        decision-making capacity, 914
    process of, 905–906, 908–912
        definition of, 910–911
        patient's psychology during,
            908–910
        surgeons' influence in, 911–912
    surrogate decisions in, 915
    with multiple physicians, 912

Institute of Medicine reports, on patient
    access, to surgical workforce, 800

Intensive care unit physician staffing, and
    better care, 884–885

Intravenous drug use, and patient
    noncompliance, 945

L

Leapfrog Group
    as health care purchasers, 883–887
    in patient safety, 874–875

Leapfrog Safe Practices Score, and better
    care, 885

Life-sustaining treatments, withdrawal of, **919–936**
case report of, 919–920, 927, 928
conflict resolution in, 930–933
difficulty with, 920
family demands for inappropriate treatment and, 930–933
legal issues in, 923–925
process of, 925–927
prognostic uncertainty and, 922–923
religious and cultural issues in, 921–922
requests for euthanasia in, 927–928
symptom control during, 928–929
in paralyzed patients, 929–930
technologic advances and, 922
variabilities in practice and, 923
versus withholding life support, 920–921

M

Medication errors, and patient safety, 871–872

Miller's pyramid, in certification for surgery, 827

Mission Cataract USA, and surgical volunteerism, 954

Morbidity and mortality conference, in patient safety, 873–874

N

National Quality Forum, in patient safety, 875

National Surgical Quality Improvement Project
in assessment of surgical care, 846–848
in patient safety, 876, 877

Negligence, definition of, 890–891

Noncompliance, and surgeons' obligations, **937–948**
alternative oaths and, 938
American College of Surgeons Code of Professional Conduct and, 940–942
American Medical Association Code of Ethics and, 939–940
definitions of noncompliance, 942–944
Hippocratic Oath and, 938
informed consent and, 941–942
prevention of noncompliance, 945–946
relevance of noncompliance, 944–945
illicit intravenous drug use and, 945
postoperative, 944–945
preoperative, 944

scope of surgeons' obligations, 938–942

O

Operation Access, and surgical volunteerism, 954

Operation Giving Back, and surgical volunteerism, 958

P

Patient safety, **867–881**
anesthesia and, 868
challenges and solutions in, 876–879
National Surgical Quality Improvement Project in, 876, 877
Quality Surgical Solutions in, 878
computerized physician order entry in, 872
crew resource management in, 870, 871
improvement of, 873–874
morbidity and mortality conference in, 873–874
simulated procedures in, 874
medication errors and, 871–872
outside influences on, 874–876
Centers for Medicaid and Medicare Services in, 875–876
Leapfrog Group in, 874–875
National Quality Forum in, 875
patient evaluation and, 868–870
postoperative care and, 871–872
surgical care processes and, 868
surgical time-out in, 870
trauma care and, 872–873

Patient Safety Indicators, in assessment of surgical care, 842

Q

Quality Surgical Solutions, in patient safety, 878

R

Residency programs, in graduate medical education, 813

Residency Review Committee for Surgery, in regulatory oversight, 815–816

Return on investment estimator, of costs and benefits, of health care, 886

S

Simulated procedures, and patient safety, 874

Surgery, new procedures and technology in, **853–866**
  credentialing and privileging in, 863–864
    American College of Surgeons and, 864
  educational interventions in, 855–862
    American College of Surgeons and, 860–861
    focus on learners, 861–862
    monitoring of outcomes, 860
    practice-based learning and improvement, 860
    preceptorship and proctoring in, 857–859
    principles and methods of, 856–857
    regional support for, 860–861
    transition to independent practice, 858–860
    variables in acquiring new skills, 857
  evidence-based information on, 854–855
  risks versus benefits of, 854

Surgery on Sundays, and surgical volunteerism, 954

Surgical care, assessing quality of, **837–852**
  American College of Surgeons in, 848
  National Surgical Quality Improvement Project in, 846–848
  outcomes in, 844–846
  Patient Safety Indicators in, 842
  processes of care in, 841–844
    Surgical Infection Prevention Project in, 842–844
  structural measures in, 838–840
    risk-adjusted mortality rates and, 839–840
    surgical volume and, 840

Surgical Council on Resident Education, and graduate medical education, 821–822

Surgical Infection Prevention Project, in assessment of surgical care, 842–844

Surgical skills laboratory, in graduate medical education, 822

Surgical volunteerism, **949–960**
  American College of Surgeons and, 957–958
    Operation Giving Back, 958
  assessing impact of, 951–952
  assessing scope of, 949–950
  educational value of, 956
  in times of disaster, 955–956

  in United States, 952–953
  innovative solutions to, 953–954
    Fresh Start Surgical Gifts, 954
    Mission Cataract USA, 954
    Operation Access, 954
    retired physicians, 954–955
    Surgery on Sundays, 954
  proven models of, 956–957
  role of surgeons in, 950–951

Surgical workforce, patient access to, **797–809**
  acute care or emergency care surgeons and, 805
  declining reimbursement and, 801–802, 804
  decrease in specialists and, 802–803
  Emergency Medical Treatment and Active Labor Act and, 803
  liability issues in, 802, 804
  physician shortage and, 800–801
    American College of Surgeons reports on, 800
    in rural areas, 801, 804
    Institute of Medicine reports on, 800
  physician supply and demand in, 797–798
    after World War II, 798
    American College of Surgeons and, 806, 808
    Bureau of Health Professions and, 798
    Council on Graduate Medical Education and, 798, 799–800, 805–806
    Flexner report and, 798
    Graduate Medical Education National Advisory Committee and, 798
    new methods of calculating, 799–800
  resident training programs in, 808
  team approach in, 807

T

Trauma care, and patient safety, 872–873

V

Volunteerism, surgical. *See* Surgical volunteerism.

W

Witnesses, expert. *See* Expert witnesses.

Moving?

Make sure your subscription moves with you!

To notify us of your new address, find your **Clinics Account Number** (located on your mailing label above your name), and contact customer service at:

E-mail: elspcs@elsevier.com

800-654-2452 (subscribers in the U.S. & Canada)
407-345-4000 (subscribers outside of the U.S. & Canada)

Fax number: 407-363-9661

Elsevier Periodicals Customer Service
6277 Sea Harbor Drive
Orlando, FL 32887-4800

*To ensure uninterrupted delivery of your subscription, please notify us at least 4 weeks in advance of move.

United States Postal Service

Statement of Ownership, Management, and Circulation
(All Periodicals Publications Except Requestor Publications)

1. Publication Title	2. Publication Number	3. Filing Date
Surgical Clinics of North America	5 2 9 - 8 0 0 0	9/14/07

4. Issue Frequency	5. Number of Issues Published Annually	6. Annual Subscription Price
Feb, Apr, Jun, Aug, Oct, Dec	6	$220.00

7. Complete Mailing Address of Known Office of Publication (Not printer) (Street, city, county, state, and ZIP+4)

Elsevier Inc.
360 Park Avenue South
New York, NY 10010-1710

Contact Person: Stephen Bushing

Telephone (Include area code): 215-239-3688

8. Complete Mailing Address of Headquarters or General Business Office of Publisher (Not printer)

Elsevier Inc., 360 Park Avenue South, New York, NY 10010-1710

9. Full Names and Complete Mailing Addresses of Publisher, Editor, and Managing Editor (Do not leave blank)

Publisher (Name and complete mailing address)

John Schrefer, Elsevier, Inc., 1600 John F. Kennedy Blvd. Suite 1800, Philadelphia, PA 19103-2899

Editor (Name and complete mailing address)

Catherine Bewick, Elsevier, Inc., 1600 John F. Kennedy Blvd. Suite 1800, Philadelphia, PA 19103-2899

Managing Editor (Name and complete mailing address)

Catherine Bewick, Elsevier, Inc., 1600 John F. Kennedy Blvd. Suite 1800, Philadelphia, PA 19103-2899

10. Owner (Do not leave blank. If the publication is owned by a corporation, give the name and address of the corporation immediately followed by the names and addresses of all stockholders owning or holding 1 percent or more of the total amount of stock. If not owned by a corporation, give the names and addresses of the individual owners. If owned by a partnership or other unincorporated firm, give its name and address as well as those of each individual owner. If the publication is published by a nonprofit organization, give its name and address.)

Full Name	Complete Mailing Address
Wholly owned subsidiary of	4520 East-West Highway
Reed/Elsevier, US holdings	Bethesda, MD 20814

11. Known Bondholders, Mortgagees, and Other Security Holders Owning or Holding 1 Percent or More of Total Amount of Bonds, Mortgages, or Other Securities. If none, check box ☐ None

Full Name	Complete Mailing Address
N/A	

12. Tax Status (For completion by nonprofit organizations authorized to mail at nonprofit rates) (Check one)
The purpose, function, and nonprofit status of this organization and the exempt status for federal income tax purposes:
☑ Has Not Changed During Preceding 12 Months
☐ Has Changed During Preceding 12 Months (Publisher must submit explanation of change with this statement)

PS Form 3526, September 2006 (Page 1 of 3 (Instructions Page 3)) PSN 7530-01-000-9931 PRIVACY NOTICE: See our Privacy policy in www.usps.com

---

13. Publication Title	14. Issue Date for Circulation Data Below
Surgical Clinics of North America	June 2007

15. Extent and Nature of Circulation		Average No. Copies Each Issue During Preceding 12 Months	No. Copies of Single Issue Published Nearest to Filing Date
a. Total Number of Copies (Net press run)		5967	5600
b. Paid Circulation (By Mail and Outside the Mail)	(1) Mailed Outside-County Paid Subscriptions Stated on PS Form 3541. (Include paid distribution above nominal rate, advertiser's proof copies, and exchange copies)	2555	2379
	(2) Mailed In-County Paid Subscriptions Stated on PS Form 3541 (Include paid distribution above nominal rate, advertiser's proof copies, and exchange copies)		
	(3) Paid Distribution Outside the Mails Including Sales Through Dealers and Carriers, Street Vendors, Counter Sales, and Other Paid Distribution Outside USPS®	1989	1776
	(4) Paid Distribution by Other Classes Mailed Through the USPS (e.g. First-Class Mail®)		
c. Total Paid Distribution (Sum of 15b (1), (2), (3), and (4))	▲	4544	4155
d. Free or Nominal Rate Distribution (By Mail and Outside the Mail)	(1) Free or Nominal Rate Outside-County Copies Included on PS Form 3541	191	165
	(2) Free or Nominal Rate In-County Copies Included on PS Form 3541		
	(3) Free or Nominal Rate Copies Mailed at Other Classes Mailed Through the USPS (e.g. First-Class Mail)		
	(4) Free or Nominal Rate Distribution Outside the Mail (Carriers or other means)		
e. Total Free or Nominal Rate Distribution (Sum of 15d (1), (2), (3) and (4))	▲	191	165
f. Total Distribution (Sum of 15c and 15e)	▲	4735	4320
g. Copies not Distributed (See instructions to publishers #4 (page #3))		1232	1280
h. Total (Sum of 15f and g)	▲	5967	5600
i. Percent Paid (15c divided by 15f times 100)		95.97%	96.18%

16. Publication of Statement of Ownership

☑ If the publication is a general publication, publication of this statement is required. Will be printed ☐ Publication not required
in the October 2007 issue of this publication.

17. Signature and Title of Editor, Publisher, Business Manager, or Owner

[signature] Joseph Fenucci – Executive Director of Subscription Services

Date: September 14, 2007

I certify that all information furnished on this form is true and complete. I understand that anyone who furnishes false or misleading information on this form or who omits material or information requested on the form may be subject to criminal sanctions (including fines and imprisonment) and/or civil sanctions (including civil penalties).

PS Form 3526, September 2006 (Page 2 of 3)